Gender, Health and Welfare

The role of gender in shaping social policy is now one of considerable interest and debate. Current controversies over the nature and funding of the welfare state have reopened historical issues. *Gender, Health and Welfare* deals primarily with the century before the creation of the classic welfare state in Britain. It provides a stimulating introduction to a historical era which saw a huge expansion in welfare services, both state and voluntary, and during which women emerged as significant 'consumers' and 'providers' of various welfare measures.

The themes covered in this book include: an introductory chapter which contextualises the volume as a whole, as well as providing a guide to the current historiographical debate; the relationship between gender and welfare in the late nineteenth and early twentieth centuries; the attitudes of the Labour Party to child welfare in the inter-war period; a critical examination of how welfare policies in both England and Japan crucially affected women's life chances; a study of the relationship between poverty, health and gender from 1870 to the inauguration of the National Health Service; case studies of the housing reformer, Octavia Hill, and the prominent female reformer, Louisa Twining; an examination of the issue of birth control in post-World War I Britain, concentrating on the successes and failures of women in the Labour movement; and a study of welfare provision for old people in Britain.

Gender, Health and Welfare discusses how, and why, gender was important in shaping modern welfare provision. The contributors – several with international reputations – address key issues which will appeal to all students on courses in social policy, gender studies and social history.

Anne Digby is Professor of Social History and **John Stewart** is Senior Lecturer in British Political History, both at Oxford Brookes University, Oxford.

Gender, Health and Welfare

Edited by Anne Digby and
John Stewart

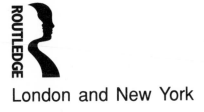

London and New York

First published 1996
by Routledge
11 New Fetter Lane, London EC4P 4EE

Simultaneously published in the USA and Canada
by Routledge
29 West 35th Street, New York, NY 10001

Typeset in Times by Florencetype Ltd, Stoodleigh, Devon
Printed and Bound in Great Britain by TJ Press (Padstow) Ltd,
Padstow, Cornwall

British Library Cataloguing in Publication Data
A catalogue record for this book is available from the
British Library

Library of Congress Cataloguing in Publication Data
A catalogue record for this book has been requested

ISBN 0–415–12886–2

Contents

List of illustrations   vii
Notes on contributors   viii
Acknowledgements   x

1 **Welfare in context**   1
  Anne Digby and John Stewart

2 **Excess female mortality: constructing survival during**
  development in Meiji Japan and Victorian England   32
  Sheila Ryan Johansson

3 **Poverty, health and the politics of gender in Britain,**
  1870–1948   67
  Anne Digby

4 **Octavia Hill and women's networks in housing**   91
  Caroline Morrell

5 **Late nineteenth-century philanthropy:**
  the case of Louisa Twining   122
  Theresa Deane

6 **The campaign for birth control in Britain in the 1920s**   143
  Lesley Hoggart

7 **'The children's party, therefore the women's party':**
  the Labour Party and child welfare in inter-war
  Britain   167
  John Stewart

8 **Gender, welfare and old age in Britain, 1870s–1940s**   189
  Pat Thane

**9 Gender and welfare in the late nineteenth and
early twentieth centuries**   208
Jane Lewis

Index   229

Illustrations

TABLES

2.1 The extent of excess female mortality in Japan, 1908,
as measured using male/female mortality ratios   37

2.2 The range of male/female life (e_0) differentials for
relatively poor, predominantly rural populations whose
overall level of female life expectancy is between
40 and 49   38

2.3 Two 'standard' patterns of male/female age-specific
death rate ratios at life expectancy at birth levels
below 45, compared to values for Japan in 1908
(with an abbreviated comparison to India, 1951–60)   40

2.4 Life expectancy at birth: males and females, Japan,
1891–1975   44

2.5 Male and female life expectancy at birth in a Hida
Prefecture Temple Death Register   45

2.6 Sex ratios for selected countries in 1975 and Japan at
various dates (total male population over total female
population)   45

2.7 Excess female mortality in Victorian England and
Meiji Japan based on male/female age-specific
mortality ratios (M/F)   55

8.1 Percentage of population aged 65 and over,
Great Britain, 1851–1981   191

FIGURE

2.1 Life expectancy advantage at birth for males and
females during development (in years)   43

Contributors

Theresa Deane is a D.Phil. student at the University of Sussex who is researching the relationship between professionalisation and nineteenth-century philanthropy, with special reference to Louisa Twining.

Anne Digby is Professor of History at Oxford Brookes University. She has written extensively on the history of social welfare and of medicine. Among her recent publications is *Making a Medical Living: Doctors and Patients in the English Market for Medicine, 1720–1911*, Cambridge, Cambridge University Press, 1994.

Lesley Hoggart is a Ph.D. student at Goldsmiths' College, University of London. She is currently completing her thesis on birth control politics in twentieth-century Britain. She then intends to do further research on abortion politics in Europe.

Sheila Ryan Johansson is a Senior Research Fellow at the Wellcome Unit for the History of Medicine, University of Oxford. As a medical demographer, she is currently investigating the connection between medical advances and improved life expectancy in the English aristocracy during the seventeenth and eighteenth centuries.

Jane Lewis is Professor of Social Policy and Administration at the London School of Economics. She has published widely on social policy and women's history. Her recent works include *Women and Social Action in Victorian and Edwardian England*, Aldershot, Edward Elgar, 1991.

Caroline Morrell is a part-time lecturer in Housing Studies in the School of Planning, Oxford Brookes University. She is currently completing a Ph.D. thesis on 'Women and the Housing Movement, 1860–1914'.

John Stewart is Senior Lecturer in British Political History, Oxford Brookes University. He has published on child welfare policy and left-wing medical politics in inter-war Britain, and is currently working on a history of the Socialist Medical Association.

Pat Thane is Professor of Contemporary History, University of Sussex. Among her many publications on the history of social welfare, women and the Labour movement are Gisella Bock and Pat Thane (eds), *Maternity and Gender Policies*, London, Routledge, 1991.

Acknowledgements

The chapters in this volume originated in a conference on 'Gender, Health and Welfare' held in the Humanities Research Centre at Oxford Brookes University, in November 1993. We should like to thank Jo Mosley for her enthusiastic organisation of the conference, Tina Duffelen and Pauline Tobin for their continuing administrative and secretarial help, and Jessica Feinstein for her technical assistance.

Chapter 1

Welfare in context

Anne Digby and John Stewart

This volume is concerned with the exploration of a number of
themes including the gendered allocation of welfare resources in
society and the role of family and state in influencing this division;
the effect of gender in the creation and adoption of policies concerning health and welfare by pressure groups, political parties,
and government at both local and national levels; and the extent
to which the balance of voluntary and statutory bodies alters the
nature of welfare, not least because of the differential involvement
of men and women. These issues involve not only structure but
agency and thus include discussions of the ways in which welfare
agendas are shaped in different contexts. A significant theme is
the role of female agency in networks during the earlier development of welfare policies and systems, while another key area of
debate is whether women should continue to be interpreted as
being primarily consumers of welfare, rather than providers/
producers/managers of welfare. These related issues give analytical coherence to an interconnected series of case studies from the
mid-nineteenth to the mid-twentieth century, which centre on
Britain within a wider international setting. This first chapter
provides a general historiographical review of British welfare
development and a discussion of the contribution that a gendered
analysis can make to it.

BEFORE THE CLASSIC WELFARE STATE

The century which ended with the creation of the 'classic' welfare
state saw a fundamental change in the role of the British state.
The mid-nineteenth century was an era of *laissez-faire* when
central government adopted a minimalist role in social and

economic affairs. In social policy, the single most important piece of legislation remained the 1834 Poor Law Act, motivated in part by Malthusian and Benthamite ideology stressing both individual moral – and thereby social and economic – responsibility and administrative efficiency. After World War II, such ideas appeared to have been discarded; the Labour government, drawing on a mixture of Keynesian economics and labourist concerns for social justice, intervened on an unprecedented scale in both economy and society. Particularly as enshrined in health provision, the stress was on universal, comprehensive and free services, stripped of the stigma associated with nineteenth-century notions of pauperism and the undeserving poor.[1]

This is a rather stark way of presenting an immensely complex period. Local bodies remained important providers of welfare, and key institutions such as the Treasury were long hostile to the kind of government expenditure which large-scale social welfare involved. Furthermore, recent work has stressed the continuing role of the non-state sector in providing welfare. This is significant for the volume of resources which the voluntary sector has, historically, distributed. In Britain, where the state has always been relatively 'weak', this is important. There is, therefore, a 'mixed economy' of welfare. Moreover, the complex relationship between the voluntary sector, the state, and society not only puts a new perspective on the state's role, it also suggests there is no 'linear' progression from the 'individualism' of the nineteenth century to the 'collectivism' of the post-World War II era. It is striking, for example, that the individual most associated with the creation of the welfare state, William Beveridge, also wrote *Voluntary Action* (1948). At a time when the impetus appeared to be towards more state direction, this work extolled the virtues of the voluntary sector even as the state appeared to be trying to take more of a role to itself.[2] A number of the contributions to this volume discuss the role of non-state welfare, for example that of Caroline Morrell on Octavia Hill and housing. When we speak of a century of dramatic change, therefore, it is not in a simplistic spirit of Whiggish interpretation of an 'inevitable' welfare state, and with it a final achievement of citizen rights. So what was it about the century after the Great Exhibition that made it so crucial in modern British social welfare history; what were the *particular* historical events and trends that led to the creation of the welfare state? Among the most important factors were: the changing intellectual climate; the influence of war; and political change, most notably the rise of Labour and the enfranchisement of women.

First, then, what changes took place in the intellectual climate?[3] If political economy dominated the mid-Victorian period, by the end of the nineteenth century there were a number of challenges to its claim to have discovered the 'natural laws' of the economy. On an empirical – but extremely important – level the findings of social investigators suggested that phenomena such as unemployment, poor housing, and the poverty of the old could not simply be explained by individual moral shortcomings. In economics, the work of Marshall questioned the tenets of classical liberal thought, while in philosophy a new, and more positive, conception of the state was emerging. In a complex way, all of these fed into the phenomenon of 'New Liberalism', an adaptation of liberal ideology which stressed a greater role for the state in social welfare matters and a more 'organic' view of society. This in turn influenced the welfare legislation of 1906 to 1914.[4] The period between the mid-nineteenth and early twentieth centuries saw, therefore, what some political scientists have described as the beginnings of the 'rise of collectivism', a point cogently made by a contemporary critic of such trends, A. V. Dicey.[5] All this is not to suggest that the key ideas of Victorian liberalism were redundant by 1914. The persistence of the 'Treasury View' in the inter-war period demonstrated the intellectual legacy of the nineteenth century, specifically regarding balanced budgets and minimum levels of public expenditure. But the era of mass unemployment, Soviet Five-Year Plans and Roosevelt's New Deal saw a continuing critique of unbridled capitalism. Keynes and Beveridge, in many respects the intellectual founders of the welfare state, are central here, although note should also be made of bodies such as Political and Economic Planning and the social democratic theorists around the Labour Party. With the success of Labour in both the wartime coalition and the 1945 election, it did at last appear as if the tenets of the 'dismal science' had been rejected, and that an era of managed, welfare capitalism had arrived.[6]

Turning now to our second general causal factor, was there, as one commentator on welfare provision has suggested, a 'close association between warfare and welfare'? From the last decades of the nineteenth century concern about the condition of the mass of the population was partly motivated by the more tense and competitive international situation.[7] Amid fears of declining relative international position and a possibly 'degenerating' race, ameliorative social policy became a major political issue, especially after the Anglo-Boer War débâcle. Like 'New Liberalism', this was to feed into the welfare reforms of 1906–14, particularly in respect of children and of health, since attention to these was perceived as potentially averting racial decline.[8] During World War I, the state took further 'collectivist' measures, and was concerned to maintain civilian morale by promises of 'reconstruction'. Although in many crucial areas such promises were not honoured, the war did raise expectations of social reform.[9] The 1920s and 1930s therefore saw an increase in social welfare provision, despite the economic constraints imposed by conventional fiscal policy. Moreover, an apparently declining population and the rise of militaristic foreign powers made health and social conditions a continuing source of concern, and it is in this context that the reports and recommendations of the 1930s, again principally about health care provision, need to be placed.[10]

What impact, then, did World War II have on the existing impetus towards social reform? This is the subject of a vigorous and ongoing historical debate. The reforming proposals and measures of the 1930s are seen by some as, effectively, constituting the welfare state in embryo, although the unplanned and uncoordinated nature of the services is generally acknowledged. Others emphasise the fundamental shift in the political mood of the period 1939–45. The welfare state was, according to this approach, very much the creation of the war itself, and increased welfare provision something advocated by all major political parties – an instance of the idea of 'convergence' in interpretations of social welfare. Others stress the novelty of Labour's post-war legislation, and the continuing hostility of the Conservatives towards comprehensively planned welfare provision. This is related to the debate over 'consensus'; whether there was a general political agreement on the aims and structures of the 'welfare state'; and whether, later on, the post-1979 Conservative administrations sought to break out of a supposedly established consensual ideological pattern.[11] What is clear is that because of the nature of the conflict, the state took control of areas of social and economic life previously deemed out of bounds. As the war progressed, there was a popular desire not to return to the 'free market' conditions of the 1930s, and, as soon as the fighting finished, for the fulfilment of the sort of welfare promises broken after 1918. The impact of the Beveridge Report of 1942 and the inclusion of the phrase 'social security' in the Atlantic Charter – a declaration of Allied War Aims – are commonly cited indicators of this groundswell of popular opinion, with the landslide victory of the Labour Party in 1945 its political expression.[12] There is thus a sound argument for seeing Britain's participation in major wars from around the late nineteenth century as important in bringing about social reform.

If changes in the intellectual climate and the impact of war were significant in setting the agenda for increased welfare provision, then it must be acknowledged that the pressures of a changing political system also had a role. The arrival of the working class on the national political stage, a process which began with the 1867 Reform Act, had at least two consequences for social policy. First, the British version of socialism was not, unlike some of its European counterparts, ever revolutionary. Instead, whatever the rhetoric, its essential aim was a better deal for the working class within capitalist society. This meant that the organised working class, and particularly in the twentieth century the Labour Party, sought economic and social reform. By World War II, Labour can be seen in important respects as the descendant of 'New Liberalism', as its acceptance of key aspects of the ideas of Keynes and Beveridge, both committed Liberals, attests.[13] In short, Labour identified itself as a party of reform, and as it rose in influence so it was able to help set the welfare agenda. Second, the reaction of other political parties to the rise of the working class also has to be taken into account. It would be wrong to see only the Labour Party as advocating social welfare. On the contrary, in the first half of the twentieth century Liberal, Conservative, Coalition and National governments all, with varying degrees of commitment, sought to address the 'condition of England' question. This was not necessarily new – nineteenth-century Tory paternalism had played an important role in social welfare provision – but was something which had moved up the political agenda, largely because of the increased weight of the working class in the national political scene.[14]

Of equal political importance is the emergence of women as participants in the political process. Most obviously, this came about with the achievement of the parliamentary franchise in 1918 and 1928, which made the major parties re-align their political strategies to take account of 'women's issues', as the chapters by Lesley Hoggart and John Stewart in this volume indicate very clearly. These frequently emphasised welfare matters. Just as significant, however, was the ability of women to vote for and be elected to various local bodies from the late 1860s onwards. This was important not least because much social welfare was provided by agencies such as Poor Law Boards of Guardians. More generally, there was a close, if complex, relationship between women's increasing participation in politics and their participation in welfare, both statutory and voluntary. In a very real sense, therefore, women were, in welfare terms, both 'consumers' and 'providers'.[15]

Women's participation in bodies such as Boards of Guardians also raises the important point of the role of local government and local institutions in British welfare provision. The development of the welfare state should not, in other words, be seen as the inexorable rise of the central state as sole welfare provider. Local agencies were key sources of welfare in the nineteenth century and if it was the case that local government was rather less independent of central government in 1914 than previously, it was also true that the range of social provision offered by the local state had increased. It was also of importance that it was in the local arena that working-class and female activists first made a political impact and, as is suggested at numerous points in this volume, social welfare was very much one of the primary concerns of each. Moreover, local welfare provision continues to have a key role. During the creation of the 'classic' welfare state, local bodies lost some functions to central government but also acquired others. This was most notably the case in respect of the post-war housing programme, secondary education, and social services. The revival of local government after World War II, a period when its very future appeared in doubt, has been attributed to Labour's strength in this area.[16]

Finally, where did Britain stand in relation to other advanced industrial countries during this period? In a stimulating chapter in this volume Sheila Ryan Johansson argues that the patriarchally oppressive policies of Meiji Japan were drawn from Victorian England's model of managing women during the process of economic development. Meiji Japan thus rejected individualism and rights for women in favour of demanding sacrifices for the sake of the nation. In post-Victorian Britain welfare services

developed only slowly in response to factors such as the enfranchisement of women, and the rise of the working class, so that it
was not until after World War II that a 'welfare state', in the sense
of centrally organised social provision, came into being. Moreover,
Britain has always had, and still retains, an important voluntary
sector, and a significant role for local government. From a long-
term perspective, therefore, Britain might be seen as a 'late' and
rather reluctant welfare state.

Germany's ideological heritage gave it few problems regarding
state intervention, and thus introduced welfare measures in the
1880s. This was an attempted 'antidote' to the rise of socialism, a
point not lost on a number of British commentators, and German
social insurance legislation influenced that of Edwardian Britain.
When introduced, the National Insurance Act of 1911 was viewed
sceptically by certain sections of the British Labour movement,
primarily because it was seen to be propping up capitalism rather
than redistributing wealth. Almost identical objections were raised
by Norwegian socialists to their country's pre-1914 welfare provisions. The complex relationship between the 'rise of labour' and
social welfare was not, therefore, confined to Britain.[17] That
welfare was truly an international and imperial issue by the end
of the nineteenth century is evident from, for example, the international conferences on labour protection and the speeches of
major politicians on the 'imperial' dimension of child welfare.[18]
This transnational dimension continued to be of significance. In
the United States the power of 'social feminists', individually and
collectively, was manifested by the passing of the 1921 Mother
and Infancy Protection Act. Moreover, these female reformers
were in close contact with their peers in Europe, suggesting that
'networks' are not confined by national boundaries. The significance of war and the consequent political emancipation of women
for societies other than Britain is also evident here. The inter-war
period saw important developments in American social welfare
policy, most famously in the 'New Deal' of the 1930s. Although
the effectiveness of its programmes remains a matter of debate,
there can be little doubt that Roosevelt's legislation marked a
significant shift in American welfare thinking. This prompted one
contemporary commentator to remark that in the decade prior to
1939 'more progress was made in public welfare and relief than
in the three hundred years after this country was settled'.
Interestingly, the New Deal programmes aroused relatively

little interest or comment in Britain.[19] Two societies which did stimulate British interest in the 1930s and 1940s, especially on the political left, were the Soviet Union and Sweden. The Soviet Union appeared to be making huge advances precisely in the era when western capitalism was on the verge of collapse, the 1930s. In the field of social welfare it had 'developed a network of services which, though still imperfect, outstripped, at least in aspiration, those of many more prosperous societies'. These achievements were enthused about by such influential British admirers of the Soviet Union as the Webbs. Social democratic Sweden, after 1932, experienced increases in public expenditure to combat unemployment and the introduction of unemployment insurance. This expansion in the welfare network was largely brought to a halt by World War II, but renewed in the immediate post-war period. After 1945 other nations also saw welfare expansion. France, for example, greatly increased its system of social insurance, part of a recognition of the need for national solidarity and social justice in the wake of unprecedented wartime upheaval. This trend was commented on at the time by the International Labour Office.[20]

Britain was not alone in creating a 'welfare state', although after 1945 it was seen as among the most comprehensive. It therefore appeared plausible that such a phenomenon was characteristic of advanced industrial societies, and that this marked an element of 'convergence' between them, irrespective of any more apparent 'ideological' difference. Such provision had arrived in societies with relatively 'weak' state apparatuses – such as Britain and the United States – as well as in those conventionally thought of as having 'strong' states – such as the Soviet Union.[21] But while the similarities between Britain and other countries have been highlighted, there were also significant differences between the ways in which welfare was individually introduced; in the balance between national and local provision; in the method of funding (whether by insurance or by general taxation); or in the relative weight assigned to statutory or voluntary agencies.

A GENDERED CONTRIBUTION TO WELFARE

The concept of a mixed economy of welfare has led historians to appreciate the changing balance between the state and voluntary sector in past welfare, and thus to a better understanding of the importance and complexity of private as well as public endeavour. Voluntarism in social welfare involved on the one hand self-help and mutual aid, and on the other charitable or philanthropic endeavour for others. Geoffrey Finlayson's perception of a Victorian emphasis on a 'citizenship of contribution' rather than the later stress on a 'citizenship of entitlement' has done much to illuminate the central significance of voluntarism and of the values that underlay it.[22] The Victorian citizenship of contribution was practised in a huge range of voluntary groups which effectively provided cradles of citizenship. Indeed it has been calculated that in England many people belonged to five or six voluntary associations, in marked contrast to France or Germany, where very few belonged to even one.[23] In this section of the chapter the relationship of female agency to voluntarism and to the developing structures of state welfare will be discussed.

'The philanthropic world was an acceptable and comfortable place for women to be',[24] and studies of the voluntary sector have given a new importance to the role of women as providers of philanthropy. Prochaska's invaluable study of Victorian philanthropy has argued that 'With a genius for fund-raising and organisation women fundamentally altered the shape and the course of philanthropy, expanding and redirecting it into channels which suited their perceptions of society and its problems.'[25] Whether as founders, managers or subscribers to charitable organisations women were thus very prominent in nineteenth-century charities.[26] Within a huge range of charitable agencies women made a significant contribution in visiting societies assisting in the relief of poverty, refuges for homeless or unprotected women, and benevolent societies for the relief of sickness or the provision of lying-in facilities. Women's contribution was distinctive in combining a growing expertise in management and a continuing personal involvement with the 'clients', so that at best they were able to impart a personal and caring character to these charitable bodies.

From a late-twentieth-century perspective there is a tendency to see these developments as purely secular activities, whereas in practice they involved moral and religious issues. This moral perspective on the relationship between the individual, society, and the state arose because it was perceived as not only what was, or would be, but what *should* be the case. It was here that the women's movement was able to play a highly significant role since women's participation in private life was conceptualised in terms of their moral contribution, and this was later used as a rationale for a more active, moral citizenship. Women used a language of service and duty to others, which equally displayed a desire to reform and change behaviour in the social territory beyond their own homes. Early voluntary work in health and welfare was linked, as Jane Lewis has observed, 'to the family and to social work performed voluntarily by middle-class women who thereby fulfilled their citizenship obligations'.[27] Victorian women's social work in housing, poor law, health, or education was performed locally, cementing links between family and community, and acting as a bridge from activist women's own families to the families of the poor whom they aimed to regenerate morally, quite as much as to help in any material or secular way. This implied for many – and certainly for the anti-suffragists who opposed a *national* vote for women – a gendered citizenship in which women emerged into the public sphere but only within the locality, either as voluntary or philanthropic workers, or within local government. In the latter they extended their influence in a public activity sufficiently limited not to contaminate the moral purity that was perceived to be the essence of the 'womanly woman', and hence the fount of feminine influence.

A local government that had been reformed and revitalised between the late 1860s and early 1890s was capable of initiating innovative policies in education, health and welfare, and this provided an opportunity for a fresh relationship between voluntary and public endeavour in the local state. Here women became active, first as members of School Boards from 1870, and then as Poor Law Guardians from 1875, before serving as councillors in what has been termed social or municipal housekeeping. Female councillors specialised in welfare areas such as the poor law, public heath, housing and education. Women councillors were much more aware of the communities in which public institutions operated and attempted to relate the two, as in the use of schools for evening community activities. Utilising expertise they acquired in voluntary charitable activities they were also more client-centred rather than using 'male' managerial skills. They 'remade the workhouse', domesticating it so that women guardians became 'surrogate mothers to pauper children, elder sisters to servant girls and unmarried mothers, and family friends to the sick and the elderly'.[28] Theresa Deane, in her chapter on Louisa Twining, notes that as Poor Law Guardian for Kensington and for Tunbridge Wells, Twining compared the workhouse to a domestic household where women should have 'a power of control'. Female councillors, as Patricia Hollis has demonstrated, thus showed equality in competence but difference in experience.[29] In the voluntary sector first-generation activists, such as Octavia Hill in housing management or Emily Davies in higher education, had earlier stressed the tactical advisability of femininity in dress and demeanour, together with more fundamentally ladylike qualities, such that the moral qualities of the private woman would result in a public good. Hill suggested, for instance, that 'a high ideal of home duty' was the best preparation for philanthropic work among the poor.[30] And in secondary education Alice Ottley commented that 'The headmistress is anxious that it should be understood that she detests women's cricket. . . . She earnestly desires that the "note" of the Worcester High School should be delicate, womanly refinement'.[31] Pioneers like these were able to subvert gendered concepts of separate spheres – where the private was perceived as female, and the public as masculine – without appearing to violate the established social order too overtly. Such social conservatism might be the product either of genuine belief or of tactical expediency, but in each case it helped to prevent a political backlash that would have impeded further advances in women's public roles.[32]

Female activity in nineteenth-century voluntary organisations has been seen as a positive achievement in the development of the welfare state through a recognition of the porous character of the boundary between the state and civil society. This, as Koven and Michel have suggested, 'could better accommodate women's historical role in state formation' and recognise female agency 'as both clients and shapers of welfare programs and policies'.[33] Feminist theorising on the welfare state has also extended the analysis beyond state and market to give greater importance to the family, and has focused more on women's dependency on men and less on dependency on the state.[34] It has recognised 'a core of commonality while paying attention to variation' between national experiences.[35]

Internationally, the extent to which early state welfare measures were directed specifically at women showed a clear bifurcation between those where measures were a supplement to those fundamentally driven by concern for an adult male labour force (as in

Britain, Germany or Scandinavia), and those where maternal provision was central (as in Italy or the USA). In America where labour legislation focused to an unusual extent on women workers, 'much of the path to the welfare state [was] blazed by middle-class women' not only because of the gender dimension but the class one also since, as has been argued controversially, 'women's activism . . . serves as a surrogate for working-class social-welfare activism'.[36] And Skocpol has suggested that 'America came close to forging a maternalist welfare state, with female-dominated public agencies implementing regulations and benefits for the good of women and children'.[37] In Italy the *cassa natisionale di maternità* of 1910 was set up thirty years after women's political engagement with the relationship between the state, motherhood and female citizenship. This enabled women factory workers to have a month off after childbirth or miscarriage, by means of tripartite payments by state, employers and workers.[38] The relationship of female gains in social rights to those in political rights was complex, since substantial gains in women's welfare could be won before the suffrage was achieved. During the 1910s and 1920s, at a time when 'mothers of the nation' did not have the right to vote in many American states, the USA came close to setting up a maternalist system of welfare; in Italy women had not got the vote by the time of the national maternity fund of 1910; and in Britain maternal and child welfare centres were well established at the local level before female suffrage was gained in 1918 and 1928. Women were thus operating in 'the interstices of political structures', and using their authority as mothers to challenge 'the constructed boundaries between public and private, women and men, state and civil society'.[39]

The 'active citizenship' that was involved in the British 'citizenship of contribution' – so characteristic of the period from the 1830s to the 1880s – was carried forward by women into the early twentieth century since, until 1928 when they gained the full adult suffrage, they were denied access to the formal entitlements of citizenship. Even when state welfare measures such as old age pensions or insurance schemes related to health and unemployment were enacted, an ethos of voluntarism favourable to female agency remained. Margaret Bondfield, the Labour Party's first female cabinet minister, was a strong supporter of contributory citizenship. In relation to the national health and unemployment schemes of 1911 she commented that:

It is a mistake to suppose that under Socialism a man is going to get all he earns. He is not. He will have to pay for the support of those who meet with accidents ... those who have reached old age ... for the very best education of the children. ... The people had to pay for this [the insurance bill], as they had to pay for everything. Some of my friends said that the Bill ought to be opposed, as it was contributory. I wanted the scheme to be contributory, so that people could see and understand the control that was in their own hands.[40]

Not that all women viewed the 1911 Act from such a gender-blind position as did Bondfield, since the Women's Industrial Council deprecated its tendency 'to consider the work of a wife and a mother in her home of no money value'.[41]

The 'male breadwinner paradigm' of the ensuing economically depressed period was highlighted by the inter-war imposition of a marriage bar in the professions, which further weakened female economic independence.[42] The dominant strand – in a woman's movement no longer united by the goal of achieving suffrage – was that of Eleanor Rathbone's 'new' or 'welfare' feminism, which advocated distinctive yet complementary roles for men and for women. In 1924 Rathbone argued that although the British women's movement had secured 'the armour of education and the weapon of political power' it 'is only beginning the most constructive and practically valuable part of its task', which was to challenge the disadvantaged economic position of women and to achieve a lessened dependence on men through family endowment (children's allowances) paid to mothers directly by the state.[43] Yet in a male-dominated central government British women achieved few successes at the national level, and had to await a post-war government for these family allowances.[44] Internationally, female progress in welfare was also chequered. In France, where pronatalist thinking was stronger than in Britain, policies targeted children directly in a more 'parental' model of social welfare; in Weimar Germany, the state's restrictive ideology articulated the needs of women in terms of motherhood; and in the USA the Sheppard-Towner Act of 1921 (that gave federal matching funds to modest state programmes to improve child and maternal health) did not survive Conservative political pressures beyond 1929.[45]

In the longer term the pace of British women's progress in advancing their welfare interests is still the subject of continuing discussion. If attention is paid less to the central than to the local state during the inter-war period it is clear that in certain localities women managed to influence the welfare agenda. Thane has argued that whereas Labour Party women nationally had a 'minimal achievement' in inter-war welfare, they had greater successes in 'persuading Labour-controlled local authorities to improve medical, maternity, and child welfare, housing, education and services such as public baths'.[46] Women might also have a more positive experience in wartime. But the degree to which governmental pronatalism and the exigencies of a labour market enabled women to work and also improved childcare facilities during wartime is debatable, since even in the 'warfare state' Summerfield has argued that a continued 'strength of patriarchal expectations' constrained women's roles.[47] A 'double helix' of gendered roles in war and peace has been suggested. In this inter-pretation the traditional roles which operated in peace were suspended in wartime, only to be curtailed in peacetime again.[48]

FORMS OF FEMALE AGENCY

Having looked at some of the achievements of women in welfare we now turn to the gendered mechanisms through which this was obtained. This section of the chapter discusses the means by which this agency operated for women in welfare through networks of friendship and association. It suggests that an analysis of the main outlines of women's contribution to welfare as producers, providers and managers will highlight a positive contribution, whose creativity and independence is intended to offset the more traditional depiction of women as dependent consumers of welfare.

A central concern of women's history has been the relationship between the public and private spheres. Prosopography (collec-tive biography) has been a useful approach in analysing the dynamics of group agency in initiating a reform or making up a welfare movement. By analysing key factors in individuals' lives pertinent common features in terms of family background, educa-tion, social or political philosophy, career aspiration or fulfilment, become highly visible. This approach was first developed in economic and political history,[49] but more recently it has been of great interest to feminist historians and to historians of social policy. It enables us to see how the profiles of different generations of women changed as historical opportunities widened. The factors that led a group of ten notable Victorian women involved in social work 'to leave their comfortable and cultivated homes, often in the face of family opposition and social disapproval, for work that was frequently physically, mentally and emotionally exhausting' has been analysed in a collective biography.[50] This enables the historian to focus on interconnections between personal experience and public personas, as in another study of five Victorian and Edwardian women. This facilitates an analysis 'of the "lived lives" of these women, [and] shows how their ideas about the proper relationships between the individual, family and the state were forged'.[51] The dilemmas caused by an apparently unproblematic victory of the suffrage being granted to women in 1918, have been illuminated in a thematic study of fourteen feminists, which included the campaigner for state-funded child allowances, Eleanor Rathbone. It showed that, with the vote, the central unifying factor in their public lives had been removed, and hence that a greater diversification of public activities in the lives of individuals – and hence in the women's movement – ensued.[52] Another larger group portrait of eighteen inter-war feminists has probed their dilemmas, choices and distinctive strategies over a longer time span. It suggests that a programme such as that of the dominant inter-war welfare feminism – which focused on child allowances and thus postulated further state interventionism in welfare – was profoundly divisive among women whose previous links had been libertarian rather than collectivist.[53]

From a greater understanding of individual women, and of the friendships that might sustain and empower them, has come a new interest in the operation of female networks in public policy. While it is clear that personal connection, often of a familial character, was important for middle-class men and women in politics, philanthropy, and academe,[54] for independent-minded women it was friendship among like-minded individuals that arguably was of the greatest importance. During the first women's movement informal connections between women possessing a common purpose constituted useful networks. These played a crucial role in a number of areas including developing secondary and higher education, advancing female suffrage, opening up new areas of employment for women, and advancing health and welfare services. Informal networks typically pooled existing knowledge among women, helped in gathering new information, furthered useful social and professional contacts, and offered invaluable emotional support in times of difficulty or doubt. Such private networking was often transitory, growing spontaneously and unself-consciously as favourable opportunities provided a fostering environment, and ceasing to exist as more apposite alternative groupings arose in response to fresh developments in the public domain.

Both male and female networks were concerned with support and, through this, with empowerment. But, in these new female networks (unlike well-established male equivalents), there was a minimal patronage element involved at first, since the objective was not so much office and influence as expanding opportunity. As women moved into public positions, however, a patronage element was introduced as different generations of women sought to 'hand on the torch' to those whom they had trained themselves. Particularly clear examples are to be found of this process in the housing and medical fields. In housing, as Caroline Morrell suggests in her chapter, Octavia Hill was 'the centre of the network of housing workers' and this resulted in a wide diffusion of the distinctive principles of her housing management. And in the medical field of general practice 'women only' practices were founded that both recruited – and were passed on to – like-minded medical women, who might be the product of the same medical school. However, it is necessary to qualify this impression of inter-generational continuity and advance since there was also a counterpoint of reaction against what was thought by an earlier generation to constitute progress in women's lives. Debates during the second half of the nineteenth century over whether legislation to protect the health of women workers was desirable,[55] or later disagreements during the 1920s and 1930s over the nature of welfare feminism,[56] indicated both considerable divergence of views and a reaction against previous ideas on how to achieve female social advancement. Central to these dilemmas was the interconnection of class and gender and a growing appreciation that female inter-ests were not monolithic but might be subject to internal tensions and strains.[57] For example, the campaigns of the Worker's Birth Control Group and the Organisation of Labour Women, discussed in Lesley Hoggart's chapter, highlighted class as well as gender in campaigning for the birth-control needs of the working-class woman.

It is useful to envisage a spectrum from formal to informal groupings in female networks. The insecurity and vulnerability of women moving into new areas of activity – often public and highly visible – meant that personal 'chains of connection' could both be a cause of initial advance and a precondition for further incremental progress. An occasion that exemplified the informal end of this spectrum was that associated with the Taunton Commission on secondary schooling in 1865, when the first women gave evidence to a public enquiry. Here the redoubtable Misses Buss, Beale and Davis attempted to alleviate each other's nervous strain by personal encouragement over a glass of claret.[58] A network that was both formal (in having a public existence), but informal (in that friendships initiated and then sustained it), was the Langham Place Circle during the 1850s and 1860s, while an example of a more formal and work-oriented network was that of the Association of Head Mistresses, founded in 1874. Within the period covered by the essays in this volume there was a range of historical contexts for networks that encompassed, on the one hand, private, personal and unofficial areas and, on the other hand, public, institutional and official ones. Female networks seem to have been more open and inclusive than male ones which, being frequently more privileged and thus with more to offer through membership, tended to be more exclusive. However, women's networks proliferated and overlapped as their public role expanded during the late nineteenth and early twentieth centuries. Those women who supported advances in secondary and higher education, for instance, formed a broader and more inclusive grouping than those who wished women to gain the national franchise. In effect women excluded themselves from such groupings on the basis of ideological conviction, rather than being excluded by others.

The networking structures used by women to advance health and welfare often showed a movement from the informal to the formal, from the voluntary to the state (whether local or central), and from those holding unpaid positions to those who were paid. Martha Vicinus' study of *Independent Women* in Britain has depicted the ways in which from 1850 unmarried women, individually and collectively, created 'new models for women's public roles', 'built institutions that grew in directions well beyond their original conception', and 'carried the utopian vision of a better world' whether as matrons in hospitals or workhouses, headmistresses or principals in schools and colleges, or working with the poor in charitable visiting societies, housing associations and women's settlements.[59] Later, a drive to develop more specialist institutional accommodation for men and women meant that female roles as 'managers' or 'providers' increased, as the distinctive needs of female inmates or clients were recognised as needing women for their administration.[60] Female-run institutions in late Victorian and Edwardian England tended to be less hierarchical, although not necessarily less authoritarian. This was not so much through any attempt to realise the rhetoric of earlier institutions that had viewed the body of inmates as a social 'family', as through a maternalist conception of the role of a female manager or provider. Thus, Theresa Deane writes of Louisa Twining as a Poor Law Guardian using a 'model of domesticity not only to expose men's inability to regulate the work of the workhouse but also to create a space for women's work as providers and managers'. And Caroline Morrell in discussing Octavia Hill's work in housing management, comments that 'the hallmark of her system was the personal and individual nature of the relationship between the lady rent-collector and the tenants'.

The discretion used by female pioneers in advancing public activity by women has helped to obscure the true extent of these advances. Indeed, the gender-blind nature of earlier studies of the welfare state[61] has meant that, until highlighted by recent feminist analysis, women were cast not in the role of producers, but rather as consumers, of welfare. A historiographical shift from viewing welfare and health provision as being formal and public services, to an acknowledgement that welfare was as much – or more – in the informal and private sectors brought a reconceptualisation of those who provided welfare.[62] Here an analysis of power resources extends beyond the state, and the operation of markets to take in the gendered division of labour between families and the state, and also that within families.[63] The important role of women as unpaid home carers for large groups of people, notably the disabled, and the frail elderly, then came into focus. While it is impossible to quantify the numbers of women involved in caring in past times, modern empirical studies have indicated that, even after public and institutional facilities had expanded, women were still the major carers of the mentally and physically handicapped. 'The major burden of care falls on women

– whether wives, mothers, spouses, siblings, or friends.'[64] For example, the family is expected to assume responsibility for the mentally impaired child and, within the family, mothers do most domestic and child-related care.[65] This was a continuation of a long tradition in familial-based care since, for instance, we know that women were prominent in the Victorian process of certifying 'idiot' children, precisely because they had been responsible for their earlier care and thus were knowledgeable about their disabilities.[66] The invisibility of carers for a long time helped to obscure the sexual division of labour in welfare and also prevented a public recognition of the carer's role. It was only in 1986, for example, that the European Court of Justice ruled that married women in Britain were entitled to receive an invalid care allowance. Earlier a convenient assumption had been that since married women were at home anyway (a presupposition increasingly falsified by employment patterns), no financial benefit was required to compensate them for their labour. In addition to the role of women as providers of care, their active role as managers and providers in philanthropy and local government, discussed above, needs to be brought into focus.

Traditionally, there has been a double standard of welfare provision for men and women.[67] Women have been heavy consumers of welfare – whether this was related to the relief of poverty or to health care needs. To some extent this was a product of their demographic profile since, living longer, they became dependent in old age. It was also a result of their relative weakness in a gender-segregated labour market. Low female earnings, and thus a low wage–benefit ratio, provided little economic incentive for women to stay off welfare benefits. But a more fundamental reason for their propensity to consume welfare was related to their customary roles in the family as mothers and as carers. A weak position in the labour market was inextricably linked to women's socially acceptable – indeed socially prescribed – role as carers of the young, the disabled, the sick and the frail elderly. Unpaid female caring itself then had a further knock-on effect on female welfare dependency in old age since, given these earlier circumstances, savings or welfare rights to pensions had been difficult to build up. The chapter by Pat Thane indicates the reasons for this in that the welfare system reproduced the gender divisions of the workforce, since in origin it aimed less to relieve poverty than to maximise work efficiency.

Cultural assumptions about femininity and masculinity thus helped to produce a distinctively gendered welfare profile. However, women as a group were less stigmatised as recipients of welfare than men, since in general their secondary status as breadwinners was recognised. The 'malingerer' or 'scrounger', who claimed welfare benefits while being capable of paid work was usually a male stereotype.[68] Female dependency linked to lack of work was criticised more selectively and infrequently. It took a period of extreme financial public stringency during the 1930s for British married women to be considered to have exploited the state insurance scheme through claiming to be unemployed or sick. Consequently, they had their right to benefits restricted.[69] Much more common has been a critical public attitude towards certain kinds of female single parenthood. Under the English poor law mothers suffered discrimination in being given indoor relief in the workhouse, as a result of having breached norms of respectability and morality through giving birth to illegitimate children.[70] And, more recently in the USA, mothers in receipt of AFDC (Aid to Families with Dependent Children), have experienced a deterioration in the real value of their welfare benefits greater than those of other groups.[71] In this context racial as well as gender stereotyping is involved, since American patterns of social welfare had developed within what was effectively a 'white men's democracy' and 'with an interweaving of race and gender' which focused on dependent – and particularly black – motherhood.[72] The contested nature of welfare politics, the gender, race and class exclusivities of welfare systems, have therefore become more visible as analytical attention has focused on power, agency and control.[73]

Welfare systems are both a product of profoundly gendered economies and themselves a means to either perpetuate or compensate for these inequities. Traditional, gender-blind analyses of the ways in which welfare systems have developed and operated have themselves helped to underpin welfare practices by sustaining stereotypes of women as dependent consumers of welfare. In contrast, feminist analysis has highlighted the ways in which welfare was oppressive to women precisely because it made patriarchal assumptions about the nature of the family, which was assumed to have been composed of a breadwinning male and a socially and economically dependent female.[74] From emphasising the discriminatory nature of welfare such analysis has developed into a more deep-seated structured view of inequalities centred around the concept of the 'family wage', where male breadwinners were paid higher wages in order to maintain dependent women and children.[75] Historical analysis of public facilities for childcare have also suggested that women have been regarded very much as a 'reserve army of labour', since childcare facilities were expanded by the state in wartime (when women's paid labour was required), and contracted in peacetime.[76] The contested nature of welfare development, in which women's concerns have been marginalised, has also received attention.[77] In this volume John Stewart's chapter suggests that although the need to appeal electorally to the newly enfranchised female was important in shaping the Labour Party's inter-war child welfare policies, nevertheless the relationship between the national party leadership and its women's organisations remained problematical, while the party's electoral propaganda was predicated on assumptions about a traditional family role for women.

The relative oppression of women's dependence on the state (through welfare), as opposed to dependence on individual men (through traditional familial structures), has also produced a thoughtful discussion.[78] The complexities of the issues when combined with the varied ideological standpoints of the analysts has produced inconclusive debate. It is recognised, however, that one paradox of the modern welfare system since the 1950s has been that, in offering employment to women, it has itself empowered women and lessened female dependency. Thus, Jane Lewis has argued that 'the development of state welfare has had the effect of drawing women into the political arena' and that 'state welfare provision becomes the cause rather than the effect of woman's agency'.[79] We now turn to look at the more recent history of that welfare provision.

AFTER THE CLASSIC WELFARE STATE

The 'classic' welfare state, defined by the Keynes/Beveridge paradigm, was in place in Britain by the middle of the twentieth century. The significance and influence of this should not be underestimated, domestically or internationally. In the former, it was to remain largely unchallenged until the economic and political crises of the 1970s. In the latter the post-1945 welfare state had a 'demonstration effect' for other countries. The Canadian welfare system, for example, was influenced – via the Marsh Report – by Beveridge.[80] From the perspective of the late twentieth century, and in the context of the issues raised in this volume, what are we to make of the creation of the 'classic' welfare state?

Despite contemporary alarms about the welfare state, it is clear that a number of its central institutions and ideas remain relatively intact. The extent to which it has suffered under the dual impact of economic recession and 'new Right' ideology is, however, a matter of debate. Some see the Keynesian dimension of the welfare state – that of demand management aimed at providing full employment – as having suffered most, but with 'New Right' leaders such as Margaret Thatcher having been incapable of more than 'marginal alterations' to welfare institutions such as social security and health provision. Others see Thatcherism as representing a more serious attack on welfare provision together with a qualitative shift in attitude towards the welfare state. Evidence cited for such a claim includes the significant rise in the 1980s of the number of children living in poverty. Similarly, there is a perception that from around 1987 – the advent of the third Thatcher administration – the emphasis shifted from a role for the state in providing services to that of financing and regulating services within a mixed economy of welfare that gave greater importance to the voluntary sector. Whatever the differences in interpretation over how the British welfare state now stands, most agree that the 'classic' welfare state was created in historical circumstances which have now passed. It was 'typical of an unusual period, perhaps never to be repeated'. This reflects, *inter alia*, a changing conception of 'the relationship between individuals and the state, and of their respective rights and responsibilities'.[81] Thus while there are widely differing explanations for the emergence of the 'classic' welfare state, there is agreement on the importance of the period from the mid-nineteenth to the mid-twentieth centuries in shaping its historical development.[82]

This is not to suggest that a group of 'perfect' welfare agencies and policies were in place in Britain by mid-century, nor that these were the product of inevitable historical evolution. As one commentator has put it, the 'kind of welfare state that developed was not, and is not, the only conceivable approach to social well-being'.[83] This more critical realisation is comparatively recent. In the immediate post-war period, historical commentaries on the origins and development of the welfare state tended to broadly accept the inevitability and desirability of state welfare provision. During the last quarter of a century, however, the welfare state has been criticised by the 'New Right', Marxists and feminists. Powerful interest groups such as the 'poverty lobby' have drawn attention to inherent flaws in existing welfare provision, and produced influential studies of continuing deprivation and unacceptable levels of poverty. What these various critiques have shown is that the 'classic' welfare state was as subject to contradictions and compromises as any other social institution. It was also the case that the post-war measures did little to 'empower' the subject in spite of contemporary beliefs about the 'fabric of citizenship'.[84] Welfare provision was not controlled directly by either the community or by individual citizens. Arguably this was particularly the case with regard to women. It has been suggested that fifty years on from Beveridge women still have not benefited significantly from the social security system; and that Beveridge successfully constructed an enduring 'ideology of womanhood' which reflects and reinforces 'the values of a patriarchal, capitalist society'. This is not universally accepted since others claim that while it may be the case that social policies have institutionalised the values prevailing in society, the welfare state has materially improved the condition of women. It has also allegedly been a focus for a critique of their overall place and role in society.[85]

This is an over-optimistic interpretation. There can be little doubt that serious gender inequalities still exist in the British welfare state, and have done so since its inception. One of the most important recent critiques of social policy has, therefore, been the attempt to apply a gendered analysis. This has included critically examining the inadequacies of previous explanations of welfare – for example by 'rereading' Titmuss.[86] Other analysts point to women's disadvantages not simply in their role as 'consumers' of welfare, but also as paid and unpaid workers without whom social services could not function. Moreover, it has tended to be men who have dominated the key professional groups within the welfare system, for example medical practitioners. It is further argued that social policy has legitimised a particular view of the family and of relationships within it, again to the disadvantage of many women. It is therefore impossible to evaluate the welfare state without understanding how it deals with women. For the welfare state 'emerged as profoundly gendered, filtering women's livelihood through the hands of men'. Furthermore, the generally subordinate experience of women is common to all social welfare regimes, national differences notwithstanding. Gender is therefore, according to such approaches, a 'central category of analysis'.[87]

The relationship of women to welfare states is, however, not simply a matter of their being systematically discriminated against in terms of benefits available, or the power structures within institutions. The activities of women in promoting social welfare, and their apparent success, have led some to point to the 'maternalist' nature of much social policy. This can be defined as involving the pursuit of, primarily, maternal and child welfare policies 'closely linked to the traditional female sphere'. In so doing, female activists moved motherhood from the private to the public sphere. This was influential in the era of welfare state formation, particularly in relatively 'weak' states, such as pre-1939 Britain, where gaps in the welfare system could be exploited. As has also been pointed out, however, maternalism, especially in Britain, is 'a highly mutable language' used to sanction welfare proposals by women and men from a range of ideological perspectives. It can therefore be argued that it 'necessarily operated in relation to other discourses – about citizenship, class relations, gender differences, and national identity, to name only a few – and in relation to a wide array of concrete social and political practices'.[88]

What this suggests is that maternalist analyses, in common with other approaches grounded in gender, have to be used with critical discrimination. Gender is not the only, or even necessarily the dominant, causal factor in *all* social policy formation. Class politics has also been very influential in the context of the rise of large working-class movements.[89] From a demographic standpoint, the family, its internal relationships, and its relationship to the state is another important dimension of welfare analysis. This has been true for the whole period of British history under consideration here, although for different reasons at different times. This is clearly illustrated by recent government policy in respect of both the old and the young, and in relation to parental responsibility. There is also a clear need here for comparative analysis, since neither continuing 'historical developments nor later divergences can be understood in the absence of such an analysis'.[90]

This first chapter has attempted both to provide a general historical context for the more detailed case studies that follow, and to signal some of the more significant and controversial issues involved in any reconceptualisation of the role of gender in the history of health and welfare. While it is clear that such policies were not gender neutral, the analyses that follow suggest that women could be privileged as well as disadvantaged. They also indicate that it is imperative to view gender within a broader counterpoint of class and age-relations. The pluralistic approach adopted in the following chapters is testimony to the significance of gender within the context of other factors in policy formation. As has been recently pointed out, the 'relationships between women and welfare, and women and state welfare, are more complicated than recent work would suggest and need to be set in a long time-frame to be appreciated'.[91] This volume is a contribution to such an understanding.

NOTES

1 On the 'classic' welfare state, see A. Digby, *British Welfare Policy*, London, Faber, 1989, ch. 4. Useful surveys of the period include D. Fraser, *The Evolution of the British Welfare State*, London, Macmillan, 2nd edn, 1984; G. Peden, *British Economic and Social Policy: Lloyd George to Margaret Thatcher*, Hemel Hempstead, Philip Allan, 2nd edn, 1991; and P. Thane, *The Foundations of the Welfare State*, London, Longman, 1982.

2 G. Finlayson, *Citizen, State, and Social Welfare in Britain 1830–1990*, Oxford, Clarendon Press, 1994, pp. 1–18, 259–60.

3 The work of J. Harris is crucial here: see, for example, her 'Political Thought and the Welfare State 1870–1940: An Intellectual Framework for British Social Policy', *Past and Present*, May 1992; 'Political Ideas and the Debate on State Welfare, 1940–45', in H. L. Smith (ed.), *War and Social Change*, Manchester, Manchester University Press, 1986; 'Victorian Values and the Founders of the Welfare State', in T. C. Smout (ed.), *Victorian Values*, British Academy and Oxford, Oxford University Press, 1992; and *Private Lives, Public Spirit: Britain 1870–1914*, Oxford, Oxford University Press, 1994, ch. 8. For a review of the methodological issues in relating intellectual trends to, *inter alia*, social policy, see M. Freeden, 'The Stranger at the Feast: Ideology and Public Policy in Twentieth Century Britain', *Twentieth Century British History*, 1990, vol. 1, pp. 9–34.

4 For further detail on these points see, for example, Peden, *British Economic*, chs 1 and 2; and A. Briggs, 'The Welfare State in Historical Perspective', *Archives Européenes de Sociologie*, 1961, vol. 2, pp. 228–46.

5 For example, W. H. Greenleaf, *The British Political Tradition: Volume 1, The Rise of Collectivism*, London, Methuen, 1983, *passim*; S. Beer, *Modern British Politics*, London, Faber, 2nd edn, 1982, ch. 3.

6 P. Clarke's *The Keynesian Revolution in the Making 1924–1936*, Oxford, Clarendon Press, 1990, is an important account of both Keynes and the 'Treasury View' in a vital period; on Beveridge, see J. Harris, *William Beveridge*, Oxford, Clarendon Press, 1977; on the vogue for planning in the 1930s, see A. Marwick, 'Middle Opinion in the Thirties: Planning, Progress and Political Agreement', *English Historical Review*, 1964, vol. LXXIX; and on the Labour Party, see S. Brooke, *Labour's War: The Labour Party During the Second World War*, Oxford, Clarendon Press, 1992.

7 Briggs, 'Welfare', p. 227; A. Marwick has been vigorous in stressing the impact of war on social policy: see, for example, *The Deluge*, Harmondsworth, Penguin, 1967; and *Britain in the Century of Total War*, Harmondsworth, Penguin, 1970. From an earlier and rather different standpoint, see also the famous and influential work by Titmuss, *Problems of Social Policy*, London, HMSO, 1950.

8 For a useful survey of the arguments and literature, see J. R. Hay, *The Origins of the Liberal Welfare Reforms*, London, Macmillan, 1975.

9 For differing interpretations of the immediate post-war period, see P. Abrams, 'The Failure of Social Reform, 1918–1920', *Past and Present*, 1963; K. Morgan, *Consensus and Disunity: The Lloyd George Coalition Government 1918–1922*, Oxford, Clarendon Press, 1979, ch. 4; and A. Marwick, 'The Impact of the First World War on British Society', *Journal of Contemporary History*, 1968, vol. 3.

10 P. Thane, 'The British Welfare State: its Origins and Character', in A. Digby and C. H. Feinstein (eds), *New Directions in Economic and Social History*, London, Macmillan, 1989, pp. 151–2. For more detail see A. Crowther, *British Social Policy 1914–1939*, London, Macmillan, 1988; and J. Stevenson, *British Society 1914–1945*, Harmondsworth, Penguin, 1984, chs 7–11.

11 These debates are reviewed in Rodney Lowe, 'The Second World War, Consensus, and the Foundation of the Welfare State', *Twentieth Century British History*, 1990, vol. 1, pp. 152–82; Finlayson, *Citizen*, pp. 253–8; D. Kavanagh, 'The Postwar Consensus', *Twentieth Century British History*, 1992, vol. 3; and P. Addison, *The Road to 1945*, London, Pimlico, rev. edn, 1994, 'Epilogue: the Road to 1945 Revisited'. The role of conflict in the health policy and the hostility of the Conservative administrations to the NHS in the post-war period is reviewed by C. Webster in, respectively: 'Conflict and Consensus: Explaining the British Health Service', *Twentieth Century British History*, 1990, vol. 1, pp. 115–51; and 'Conservatives and the Consensus: the Politics of the National Health Service, 1951–1964', in A. Oakley and A. Susan Williams (eds), *The Politics of the Welfare State*, London, UCL Press, 1994.

12 Brooke, *Labour's War*; Addison, *Road*.

13 Brooke, *Labour's War*, chs 4 and 6.

14 In the area of unemployment – increasingly identified as a major social problem from the end of the nineteenth century – see K. Brown, *Labour and Unemployment 1900–1914*, Newton Abbot,

David & Charles, 1971; and J. Harris, *Unemployment and Politics: A Study in English Social Policy 1886–1914*, Oxford, Clarendon Press, 1972. For health see C. Webster, 'Labour and the Origins of the National Health Service', in Nicolaas Rupke (ed.), *Science, Politics and the Public Good*, London, Macmillan, 1988.

15 Examples of the activism of working-class women can be found in C. Collette, *For Labour and for Women*, Manchester, Manchester University Press, 1989, ch. 3; P. Thane, 'Visions of Gender in the Making of the British Welfare State', in G. Bock and P. Thane (eds), *Maternity and Gender Policies: Women and the Rise of the European Welfare States, 1880s–1950s*, London, Routledge, 1991; and P. Graves, *Labour Women*, Cambridge, Cambridge University Press, 1994.

16 P. Thane, 'Government and Society in England and Wales, 1750–1914', and J. Harris, 'Society and the State in Twentieth-Century Britain', in F. M. L. Thompson (ed.), *The Cambridge Social History of Britain*, vol. 3, Cambridge, Cambridge Universtiy Press, 1990, pp. 47, 98.

17 E. P. Hennock, *British Social Reform and German Precedents*, Oxford, Clarendon Press, 1987, pp. 63, 152ff; Thane, *Foundations*, pp. 122–3. See also Briggs, 'Welfare', p. 247.

18 S. Rowbotham, 'Interpretations of Welfare and Approaches to the State, 1870–1920', in Oakley and Williams, *Politics*, pp. 25–8; J. Stewart, 'Children, Parents, and the State: The Children Act, 1908', *Children and Society*, 1995, p. 5.

19 M. Cohen and M. Hanagan, 'The Politics of Gender and the Making of the Welfare State: a Comparative Perspective', *Journal of Social Policy*, 1991, p. 473; quoted in James T. Patterson, *America's Struggle Against Poverty, 1900–1985*, Cambridge, Mass., Harvard University Press, 1986, p. 56; B. C. Malament, 'British Labour and Roosevelt's New Deal: the Response of the Left and the Unions', *Journal of British Studies*, 1978.

20 Thane, *Foundations*, pp. 271, 272–3; J.-P. Rioux, *The Fourth Republic 1944–1958*, Cambridge/Paris, Cambridge University Press, 1987, pp. 78–80; Briggs, 'Welfare', p. 224.

21 For an introduction to the theoretical issues, see R. Mishra, *Society and Social Policy*, London, Macmillan, 2nd edn, 1981, ch. 3. See also G. V. Rimlinger, *Welfare Policy and Industrialisation in Europe, America, and Russia*, New York, John Riley, 1971.

22 Finlayson, *Citizenship, State*, pp. 6, 8–9.

23 Harris, *Private Lives, Public Spirit*, p. 220.

24 J. Lewis, *Women and Social Action in Victorian and Edwardian England*, 1991, Brighton, Wheatsheaf, p. 303.

25 F. Prochaska, *Women and Philanthropy in Nineteenth-century England*, 1980, Oxford, Clarendon Press, p. 223.

26 Prochaska, *Philanthropy*, appendices I–IV.

27 Lewis, *Women and Social Action*, p. 1.

28 P. Hollis, *Ladies Elect. Women in Local Government, 1865–1914*, Oxford, Clarendon Press, 1987, pp. 284–5.

29 Hollis, *Ladies Elect*, pp. 391, 463, 466–8, 472; P. Hollis, 'Women in

Council: Separate Spheres, Public Space', in J. Rendall (ed.), *Equal or Different. Women's Politics, 1800–1914*, Oxford, Blackwell, 1987, p. 210.

30 O. Hill, *Our Common Land*, London, Macmillan, 1877, p. 25.

31 M. E. James, *Alice Ottley. First Headmistress of the Worcester High School for Girls*, London, Longman, 1914, pp. 98–9.

32 A. Digby, 'Victorian Values and Women in Public and Private', in Smout (ed.), *Victorian Values*.

33 S. Koven and S. Michel, 'Gender and the Origins of the Welfare State', *Radical History Review*, 1989, vol. 43, p. 113.

34 L. Bryson, M. Bittman and S. Donath (eds), 'Men's Welfare State, Women's Welfare State: Tendencies to Convergence in Practice and Theory?' in D. Sainsbury (ed.), *Gendering Welfare States*, London, Sage, 1994, pp. 118–19.

35 H. Land, 'Introduction' to special issue on 'Motherhood, Race and the State in the Twentieth Century', *Gender and History*, 1992, vol. 4, p. 285.

36 A. Kish Klar, 'The Historical Foundations of Women's Power in the Creation of the American Welfare State, 1830–1930', in S. Koven and S. Michel (eds), *Mothers of a New World*, Routledge, London, 1993, p. 44.

37 T. Skocpol, *Protecting Soldiers and Mothers. The Political Origins of Social Policy in the United States*, Cambridge, Mass., Harvard University Press, 1992, pp. 2, 529.

38 A. Buttafuoco, 'Motherhood as a Political Strategy: the Role of the Italian Women's Movement in the creation of the *cassa natisionale di maternità*', in Bock and Thane (eds), *Maternity and Gender*.

39 S. Koven and S. Michel, 'Womanly Duties: Maternalist Politics and the Origins of Welfare States in France, Germany, Great Britain and the United States, 1880–1920', *American Historical Review*, 1990, vol. 95, pp. 1077–9.

40 M. Bondfield, *A Life's Work*, Hutchinson, London, 1948, p. 358.

41 Quoted in J. Lewis and D. Piachoud, 'Women and Poverty in the Twentieth Century', in C. Glendinning and J. Millar (eds), *Women and Poverty in Britain*, London, Harvester, 1987, p. 44.

42 S. Pedersen, 'The Failure of Feminism in the Making of the British Welfare State', *Radical History Review*, 1989, vol. 43.

43 E. Rathbone, 'The Future of the Women's Movement', in G. E. Gates (ed.), *The Woman's Year Book, 1923–4*, London, NUSEC, 1924, pp. 27–9; H. Land, 'Eleanor Rathbone and the Economy of the Family', in H. L. Smith (ed.), *British Feminism in the Twentieth Century*, Aldershot, Elgar, 1990, p. 105.

44 Bock and Thane, *Maternity*, p. 114; A. Digby, 'Medicine and the State, 1900–1948', in S. Green and J. Whiting (eds), *The Boundaries of the Modern State*, forthcoming, Cambridge, Cambridge University Press, 1996.

45 S. Pedersen, *Family, Dependence, and the Origins of the Welfare State. Britain and France, 1914–1945*, Cambridge, Cambridge University Press, 1993; C. Usbourne, *The Politics of the Body in Germany:*

Reproductive Rights and Duties, London, Macmillan, 1992; M. Ladd-Taylor, 'Why does Congress wish Women and Children to Die?: the Rise and Fall of Public Maternal and Infant Health Care in the United States, 1921–1929', in V. Fildes, L. Marks, and H. Marland (eds), *Women and Children First. International Maternal and Infant Welfare, 1870–1945*, London, Routledge, 1992.

46 P. Thane, 'The Women of the British Labour Party and Feminism, 1906–45', in Smith (ed.), *British Feminism*, p. 140; P. Thane, 'Visions of Gender in the Making of the British Welfare State: the Case of Women and the British Labour Party and Social Policy, 1906–1945', in Bock and Thane, *Maternity*, p. 106.

47 P. Summerfield, *Women Workers in the Second World War. Production and Patriarchy in Conflict*, Routledge, London, 1984, pp. 190–1.

48 M. Higonnet *et al.* (eds), *Behind the Lines. Gender and the Two World Wars*, New Haven, Yale University Press, 1987.

49 L. Stone, 'Prosopography', *Daedalus*, 1971, vol. 100, p. 47.

50 J. Parker, *Women and Welfare. Ten Victorian Women in Public Social Service*, London, Macmillan, 1988, p. 2. (The ten were Florence Nightingale, Agnes Jones, Louisa Twining, Mary Carpenter, Elizabeth Fry, Octavia Hill, Beatrice Webb, Josephine Butler, Annie Besant, and Frances Power Cobbe.)

51 Lewis, *Women and Social Action*, p. 1. (The five case studies were of Octavia Hill, Beatrice Webb, Helen Bosanquet, Mary Ward and Violet Markham.)

52 J. Alberti, *Beyond Suffrage: Feminists in War and Peace, 1914–1928*, London, Macmillan, 1984. (The fourteen women in the study are Margery Corbett Ashby, Kathleen Courtney, Eva Hubback, Catherine Marshall, Emmeline Pethick Lawrence, Eleanor Rathbone, Lady Rhondda, Elizabeth Robins, Maude Royden, Evelyn Sharpe, Mary Sheepshanks, Mary Stocks, Ray Strachey and Helena Swanwick.)

53 B. Harrison, *Prudent Revolutionaries. Portraits of British Feminists between the Wars*, Oxford, Clarendon Press, 1987, p. 313.

54 N. Annan, 'The Intellectual Aristocracy', in J. H. Plumb (ed.), *Studies in Social History. A Tribute to G. M. Trevelyan*, reprint, New York, Books for Libraries Press, 1969.

55 P. Levine, *Victorian Feminism, 1850–1900*, London, Hutchinson, 1987, ch. 5, *passim*.

56 O. Banks, *Faces of Feminism. A Study of Feminism as a Social Movement*, Oxford, Blackwell, 1986, ch. 9, *passim*.

57 B. Caine, *Victorian Feminists*, Oxford, Clarendon Press, 1992, p. 242; A. Phillips, *Divided Loyalties. Dilemmas of Sex and Class*, London, Virago, 1987.

58 J. Kamm, *Hope Deferred. Girls' Education in English History*, London, Methuen, 1965, p. 205.

59 M. Vicinus (ed.), *Independent Women. Work and Community for Single Women, 1850–1920*, London, Virago, 1985, pp. 7, 292.

60 For example, L. Zedner, *Women, Crime and Custody in Victorian England*, Oxford, Clarendon Press, 1991, p. 293.

61 L. Gordon, 'The New Feminist Scholarship on the Welfare State', in L. Gordon (ed.), *Women, the State and Welfare*, Madison, University of Wisconsin Press, 1990, p. 10.
62 H. Rose, 'Rereading Titmuss: The Sexual Division of Welfare', *Journal of Social Policy*, 1981, vol. 10, pp. 493–4.
63 A. S. Orloff, 'Gender and the Social Rights of Citizenship: the Comparative Analysis of Gender Relations and Welfare States', *American Sociological Review*, 1993, vol. 58, p. 313.
64 G. Parker, 'Who Cares? A Review of Empirical Evidence from Britain', in R. E. Pahl (ed.), *On Work. Historical, Comparative and Theoretical Approaches*, Oxford, Blackwell, 1988, p. 506; S. Ayer and A. Alaszeweski, *Community Care and the Mentally Handicapped*, 1984, pp. 125, 150; P. White, *One in a Hundred. A Community Based Mental Handicap Project*, 1984, p. 2.
65 Parker, 'Who Cares?', pp. 497–8, 501–6.
66 D. Wright, ' "Childlike in his Innocence": Lay Attitudes to "Idiots" and "Imbeciles" in Victorian England', in D. Wright and A. Digby (eds), *Historical Perspectives on People with Learning Disabilities*, forthcoming, Routledge, 1996.
67 Gordon, 'Feminist Scholarship', p. 11.
68 A. Deacon, *In Search of the Scrounger*, 1976; A. Deacon and J. Bradshaw, *Reserved for the Poor*, Oxford, Blackwell, 1983.
69 J. Lewis, 'Dealing with Dependency: State Practices and Social Realities, 1870–1945', in J. Lewis (ed.), *Women's Welfare/ Women's Rights*, 1983, London, Croom Helm, pp. 27–8.
70 P. Thane, 'Women and the Poor Law in Victorian and Edwardian England', *History Workshop*, 1978, pp. 29–51.
71 Digby, *British Welfare Policy*, p. 17.
72 G. Mink, 'The Lady and the Tramp: Gender, Race, and the Origins of the American Welfare State', in Gordon, *Women, the State and Welfare*, pp. 93, 114.
73 C. Pateman, *The Sexual Contract*, Cambridge, Polity Press, 1988.
74 G. Pascall, *Social Policy: A Feminist Analysis*, London, Tavistock, 1986; E. Wilson, *Women and the Welfare State*, London, Tavistock, 1977.
75 H. Land, 'The Family Wage', *Feminist Review*, 1980, vol. 6, pp. 55–77.
76 D. Riley, 'The Free Mothers: Pronatalism and Working Mothers in Industry at the End of the Last War in Britain', *History Workshop Journal*, 1981, vol. 11.
77 A. Digby, 'Medicine and the State, 1900–1948' (see note 44).
78 H. M. Hermes, 'Women and the Welfare State: the Transition from Private to Public Dependence' and A. Borchast and B. Sim, 'Women and the Advanced Welfare State', in A. Showstack Sassoon (ed.), *Women and the State. The Shifting Boundaries of the Public and the Private*, London, Hutchinson, 1987.
79 'Gender, the Family and Women's Agency in the Building of "Welfare States": the British case', *Social History*, 1994, vol. 19, p. 55.
80 R. Mishra, *The Welfare State in Capitalist Society*, Hemel Hempstead, Harvester Wheatsheaf, 1990, p. 6.
81 Mishra, *Welfare State*, pp. 116–17; 'Social Policy in the Postmodern

World', in C. Jones (ed.), *New Perspectives on the Welfare State in Europe*, London, Routledge, 1993, pp. 18–19, 24–5; C. Offe, *Contradictions of the Welfare State*, London, Hutchinson, 1984, pp. 152–3; R. Lowe, 'The Welfare State in Britain since 1945', *ReFRESH*, 1994, vol. 18, p. 2; A. Oakley, 'Introduction', and R. Lowe, 'Lessons from the Past: the Rise and Fall of the Classic Welfare State in Britain, 1945–1976', in Oakley and Williams (ed.), *Politics*; J. Krieger, 'Social Policy in the Age of Reagan and Thatcher', in R. Miliband, L. Panitch, J. Saville (eds), *Socialist Register 1987*, London, Merlin Press, 1987, pp. 182, 196.

82 For a useful introduction to these, see P. Flora and A. J. Heiden-heimer, 'The Historical Core and Changing Boundaries of the Welfare State', in P. Flora and A. J. Heidenheimer, *The Development of Welfare States in Europe and America*, New Brunswick and London, Transaction Books, 1981.

83 S. Rowbotham, 'Interpretations', in Oakley and Williams (ed.), *Politics*, pp. 34–5.

84 P. Thane, 'The Historiography of the British Welfare State', *Social History Society Newsletter*, Spring 1990, vol. 15, no. 1, pp. 12–15; see also the comments on A. Briggs, one of the historians to first take a serious interest in the history of the welfare state, in D. Cannadine, 'Welfare State History', in *The Pleasures of the Past*, Glasgow, Fontana, 1988; for a brief exposition of recent critiques of the welfare state, see R. Lowe, 'Postwar Welfare', in P. Johnson, *Twentieth Century Britain*, 1994, London, Longman, pp. 370ff; Briggs, 'Welfare State', p. 227.

85 J. Colwill, 'Beveridge, Women and the Welfare State', *Critical Social Policy*, 1994, 41, pp. 53–4; R. Lowe, *The Welfare State in Britain since 1945*, London, Macmillan, 1993, pp. 33–7.

86 Rose, 'Rereading Titmuss.' Note, however, that Rose is concerned also to point to the strengths of 'traditional' approaches to welfare, and to the problems, at least at the time of writing, of 'grasping theoretically the specific position of women within both the domestic and the socialised sectors of welfare': p. 501.

87 J. Dale and P. Foster, *Feminists and State Welfare*, London, Routledge, 1986, pp. ix, 9; Pascall, *Social Policy*, pp. 1,8; Pedersen, 'The Failure of Feminism', p. 104; M. Langan and I. Ostner, 'Gender and Welfare: Towards a Comparative Framework', in G. Room (ed.), *Towards a European Welfare State?*, Bristol, School for Advanced Urban Studies, 1991; R. Moeller, 'The State of Women's Welfare in European Welfare States', *Social History*, 1994, p. 393.

88 Koven and Michel, *Mothers of a New World*, pp. 2, 125; Koven and Michel, 'Gender and the Origins', p. 115.

89 See the comments of G. Esping-Andersen and W. Korpi, 'Social Policy as Class Politics in Post-War Capitalism: Scandinavia, Austria, and Germany', in J. H. Goldthorpe (ed.), *Order and Conflict in Contemporary Capitalism*, Oxford, Clarendon Press, 1984, p. 179.

90 Pedersen, *Family, Dependence*, p. 12.

91 Lewis, 'Gender, the family and women's agency', p. 55.

Chapter 2

Excess female mortality
Constructing survival during development in Meiji Japan and Victorian England[1]

Sheila Ryan Johansson

THE POLITICAL ECONOMY OF MORTALITY

It has been estimated that there may be as many as 100 million adult women 'missing' from the world's censuses,[2] largely because so many females died prematurely while young (not because so many adult women die in childbirth).[3] Those missing women come from developing countries like India, Pakistan and China, a fact which creates the impression that excess female mortality among children is something foreign to the European cultural tradition. But it is not. Developing Europe, including Victorian England, was once characterised by pervasive excess female mortality in childhood,[4] and so was developing Japan.

No one has ever estimated how many females died prematurely during the nineteenth and early twentieth centuries in either Western Europe or Japan, probably because measuring the magnitude of excess female mortality involves basic conceptual and data problems that only become more difficult as they become historical, and data quality problems naturally arise.[5] But in either the past or the present the greatest challenge remains explaining why females should die at higher rates than males, especially as children and adolescents, in any place or time.

Explanations for any kind of differential mortality generally sort themselves into those which treat mortality as if it were a biological phenomenon expressed independently of any cultural considerations, and those which integrate biological constraints on survival with the social construction of human responses to disease environments.[6] While childbearing might be considered a natural biological hazard, excess female mortality in childhood and early adolescence is not caused by pregnancy or childbirth.[7] Moreover, while high fertility populations might be expected to have excess female mortality among adult women younger than 45 years of age, many do not.

These facts suggest that narrowly biological considerations are insufficient to explain excess female mortality. Instead it may involve the way gender was socially constructed by countries experiencing development. Indeed it is possible that excess female mortality was partly constructed by governments through the reforms they did or did not adopt in connection with it, and the changes they did or did not make in the traditional 'status' of women.

Economists who study excess female mortality among young girls routinely ignore policy issues to focus on differential labour force participation as the explanation for excess female mortality. Where daughters cannot find paid employment, but sons can, boys are more valuable to their parents, especially when daughters must be given dowries at marriage. Faced with limited incomes most parents rationally allocate scarce resources to favour the health and well-being of sons, thus investing in the children most likely to produce income for the household.[8] Once married, mothers who are dependent on sons for old age security will perpetuate the cycle of under-investing in their own daughters in order to improve their chances of a secure old age.[9]

What the sociological perspective adds to an economic story about adults (male or female) rationally pursuing their self-interest at the household level is the idea that expensive daughters and dependent widows are themselves cultural constructs. They are a reflection of institutionalised values and norms about chastity, family honour and marriage which make girls into children who cannot be given the right to work, and wives into adults who have no control over resources other than through their adult sons.[10] Thus, sociologists who study excess female mortality on the Indian subcontinent see labour market inequality as a by-product of patriarchal traditions which strictly limit the freedom of both young girls and adult women, and which encourage the assignment of a lesser value to female life.[11]

The importance of socially attaching a lower value to female life is underlined by the fact that some areas of South Asia have excess female mortality, despite the fact that young girls and adult women do work for wages.[12] Nevertheless the distribution of health-related resources within the family is still skewed towards males, and excess female mortality persists. In general, sociologists argue that the more culturally patriarchal the area in India, the more excess female mortality can be found, especially during childhood.[13]

In short, sociologically oriented approaches to the explanation of excess female mortality assume that deeply ingrained values, norms and customs create standardised patterns of biased choice within households, with or without reinforcement from biased labour markets.[14] But the stress placed by sociologists on the importance of value systems stops short of examining the role played by governments (national and local) in strengthening or undermining the institutions and behaviours associated with patriarchy, particularly during the new conditions created by development.

Governments always have the option of supporting or undermining traditional value systems through policy, in particular through institutional reforms which create or destroy the incentive systems to which ordinary people respond in the course of their daily lives.[15] Incentives can be used to change or reinforce the norms for acceptable or unacceptable behaviour, including labour market behaviour as well as health-related behaviour. The institutionalisation of incentives can increase or decrease the probability that certain individual choices will both be made and rewarded in communities, labour markets and households, especially during periods of rapid change. Formal political institutions also discourage deviance by detecting and punishing unwanted expressions of individual choice. Even more importantly institutions can give or take away basic human rights, rights that play a role in preserving health, combating disease, and preventing premature death, in the home or the workplace. From this perspective it is possible to argue that government policy can be a life and death matter.[16]

When governments and their policies are used to explain the incentives which influence individual choice, either in households or labour markets, a political economy approach is being used to synthesise some of the insights of both economists and sociologists.[17] This approach was a familiar one to political philosophers of the ancient East. In the fifth century before the common era a Chinese king (King Hu of Leang) asked to receive instruction from the philosopher Mencius. Mencius asked him: 'Is there any difference between killing a man with a stick and killing a man with a sword?' The king replied that there was no difference.

Mencius then asked: 'Is there any difference between killing a man with a sword and killing a man with a system of government?' The king conceded that there was none.[18]

Presumably governments can kill women as well as men. In connection with excess female mortality, the political economy approach asks us to consider how government policies might have influenced the construction of gender during the process of development, in a way that made it temporarily hazardous to be a young female during a period of accelerated social and economic change. This is not an easy question to answer, because government policy comes in so many forms, all of which can have both intended and unintended effects on ordinary people, including their health and survival.

THE STATE AND MORTALITY DURING DEVELOPMENT

That state policy had wide-ranging influences on survival has been recognised by Western political economists since the enlightenment.[19] Today only those economists who refuse to consider their subject 'power neutral' [20] continue to explore the politics of health and mortality.[21] Comparatively few sociologists have tried to estimate the impact of government behaviour on human behaviour related to health and mortality, possibly because health systems themselves are so often thought of as having developed over time under historically unique circumstances independent of government policy.[22] Nevertheless, it is obvious that government influence can be deployed to either reduce the extent of premature death or increase it. During development most governments explicitly adopted policies intended to prevent premature death, especially among young males and females, by reducing the extent of epidemic disease. When efficiently enforced, these public health policies can be made to work. Some demographers argue that they are the principal reason for the rise of life expectancy in modern developing countries.[23] But the state can also adopt pernicious and violent policies, including those which classify certain populations as expendable. The twentieth century has been 'distinguished' by a number of governments which have used their powers to start wars and/or conduct campaigns designed to eradicate deviants, dissidents or defectives, the Holocaust being the most tragic example.

While no modern government ever adopted explicit policies designed to produce excess female mortality, some social scientists are now beginning to explore how they might have done so implicitly,[24] through a wide range of policies which have indirect or unintended consequences for female health and mortality, particularly at the household level.[25] Implicit anti-natal policies with respect to fertility are those policies which raise the cost of children to married couples or single women, and thereby reduce or increase the willingness to have them, irrespective of what the intentions of governing élites may have been with respect to promoting population growth through explicit policies intended to keep fertility high. Thus a policy which adopts and enforces compulsory schooling and restricts child labour may reduce fertility, even if the state did not intend such a policy to have that effect. It is the absence of deliberate intention on the part of a government which makes a policy implicit rather than explicit.

After 1868 the reforming Meiji government began a sweeping campaign to initiate economic development along Western lines.[26] The campaigns involved gradually refining a series of policies intended to give both sexes a specific role in the development process. Some of these formal policies have already been identified by historians as having a profound impact on the relative welfare of women, although not necessarily on their mortality.[27] Few governments have ever been as able or as willing to impose their will at the local level as effectively as Japan during the late nineteenth and early twentieth centuries.[28] Local officials, selected for their dedication to the government's reforms, were expected to enforce all the government's policies efficiently, using the rural and urban police force to ensure local compliance when necessary. The police were empowered to inspect private dwellings to make sure that they were cleaned properly once a year, and that every household had an altar to the emperor. In this political climate failure to conform became difficult and socially costly for both men and women. Because the police brought the government's presence into the home, historians try to see how it touched individual lives.[29] In this chapter we shall consider how the government's new policies could have so compromised the relative welfare of young girls and young women that it shortened the lives of a substantial number, during infancy, childhood, adolescence as well as the reproductively active years.

Attention must be paid, first, to what excess female mortality means and, second to the specific pattern that excess female mortality took in Japan during the first half-century of development. Next Japan will be compared to other developing countries like Victorian Britain, late nineteenth-century America, as well as mid-twentieth-century India.

MEASURING EXCESS FEMALE MORTALITY

At the turn of the twentieth century males and females in Japan had the same level of life expectancy at birth (43 years); but that apparent equality concealed a pattern of age-specific death rates for females which were absolutely higher than those of same age males from very early childhood through mid-life. Table 2.1 uses male/female mortality ratios in 1908 to show how much higher (in percentage terms) female death rates were than male death rates after about four decades of economic and social development.

Table 2.1 The extent of excess female mortality in Japan, 1908, as measured using male/female mortality ratios

Age	Group	Male : Female mortality ratio	Per cent advantage
0–1	Infancy	112	12% more males die
1–4	Childhood	96	4% more females die
5–9		92	8% more females die
10–14	Adolescence	68	33% more females die
15–19		74	26% more females die
20–24	Marriage and children	73	27% more females die
25–29		67	33% more females die
30–34		74	26% more females die
35–39		79	21% more females die
40–44		95	5% more females die
45–49	Menopause	113	13% more males die
50–54		126	26% more males die
55–59	Retirement	129	29% more males die
65–69	Widowhood	114	14% more males die
70–74		107	7% more males die

Source: S. H. Preston, N. Keyfitz and R. Schoen, *Causes of Death. Life Tables for National Populations*, New York, 1972, pp.420–2. See the M_x column.

While these observed differences in age-specific death rates can be considered 'biological', none can be traced to exclusively genetic considerations which are beyond societal influence.[30] Since Japan was a very poor country in 1908, it is natural to assume that excess female mortality might have reflected this poverty, as well as the demographic fact that life expectancy at birth was still low by modern standards. That is why it is important to consider the comparative data in Table 2.2.

Table 2.2 contains a selection of low-income, low-life-expectancy societies, whose populations were predominantly rural, like that of Japan in 1908. As a whole, the selected countries demonstrate that diverse demographic outcomes are possible, even in adverse circumstances, and that excess female mortality is not a necessary correlate of either pervasive poverty, low life expectancy, or rural life. Some countries have excess female mortality and some do not, which leaves room for the possibility

Table 2.2 The range of male/female life (e_0) differentials for relatively poor, predominantly rural populations whose overall level of *female* life expectancy is between 40 and 49

Country	Date	Income level	Life expectancy at birth Male	Female	Difference	Date
India	1967	67	48.9	46.2	−2.7	1966–70
Cambodia	1958	74	44.2	43.3	−0.9	1958–9
Japan	1897–8	68	44.0	44.4	+0.4	1899–1903
Philippines	1938	68	44.8	47.7	+2.9	1938
Sweden	1816–40	'low'	39.5	43.6	+4.1	1816–40
United Arab Emirates	1939	60	35.7	41.5	+5.8	1936–8
Higher income similar level of life expectancy						
Italy	1899–1908	226	44.2	44.5	+0.3	1901–11
Spain	1906–13	225	40.9	41.7	+1.8	1910

Source: With the exception of Sweden, the income data (standardised to 1963 US dollars) and the life expectancy data comes from S. H. Preston's *Mortality Patterns in National Populations*, New York, Academic Press, 1976, pp. 34–6. Sweden's national per capita income in 1816–40 (expressed in terms of 1963 US dollars) is not available. It was probably higher than that of the other, largely Asian countries incuded in the table. But Italy and Spain are also included to demonstrate that higher levels of income alone do not necessarily produce Sweden's more favourable patterns of sex differentials, even among predominantly rural countries in a European context.

that the observed mortality ratios are a socially constructed outcome to some extent, not an outcome imposed by biological circumstances beyond a government's control.

We can ask, nevertheless, how common or uncommon excess female mortality is among poor, rural countries which have low levels of life expectancy at birth. This is another way of asking how typical or atypical Japan might have been, given its general circumstances. Samuel Preston provided one answer to that question in his 1976 study. He used virtually all the high-quality mortality data available for low-life-expectancy countries. First he averaged their age-specific death rates to create a standard set of rates for males and females sharing an overall level of life expectancy.[31] Next he identified those countries in which females had an above or below average mortality advantage. Using these methods Preston measured what amounted to relative excess female mortality. Those countries with absolute excess female mortality (i.e. where females die at a higher rate than males over some specified age or ages) are a subset of this larger set of countries.

Using Preston's data for low-life-expectancy populations, Japan's women still come out as distinctly disadvantaged, although they are not as badly off as females in India in the middle of the twentieth century.

In Table 2.3 Japan's 1908 male/female mortality ratios are compared to what can be called the Preston standard, and to a population which can be said to have set the highest historical standard for women in poor, low-life-expectancy rural populations – Sweden in the mid-nineteenth century, a country still a few decades from its own drive for economic development. For 100 years prior to this time in Sweden's history there was no absolute excess female mortality at any age, despite extensive rural poverty and a very harsh climate. It is interesting to note that despite differences in the average age of marriage, married women in each country had between five and six births before completing fertility. But there is no absolute excess female mortality during the childbearing years in Sweden; nor is there any absolute excess in the Preston standard, despite the diversity of cultures it encompasses.

More interesting still are the male/female mortality ratios for infants.[32] In Sweden female infants out-survive male infants by 18 per cent. The Preston standard is just a little lower. But Japanese female babies have only a 12 per cent advantage, a value which

Table 2.3 Two 'standard' patterns of male/female age-specific death rate ratios at life expectancy at birth levels below 45, compared to values for Japan in 1908 (with an abbreviated comparison to India, 1951–60)

Age group	The Swedish standard (1841–51)	The Preston standard 19th–20th century	The Japanese values for 1908	India (1951–60)
0 Youth	118	116	112	108
1	110	97	96	94
5	104	94	92	
10	105	87	67	102 (5–14)
15	101	92	74	
20	124	100	73	65 (15–24)
25 Marriage and	127	100	67	
30 child-bearing	124	103	74	65 (25–34)
35	131	107	79	
40	137	123	95	107 (35–44)
45	151	130	113	
50 Old age	145	131	126	162 (45–54)
55	136	129	129	
60	126	121	131	152 (55–64)
65	123	117	114	
70	114	113	107	133 (65+)
75	112	109	106	
80	114	108	104	
Life expectancy at birth:	M=40 F=44	Both sexes below 45	M=43.4 F=43.5	M=41.9 F=40.5

Sources:
1 Sweden: see G. Sundbarg, *Bevolkerungsstatistik Schwedens, 1750–1900,* Urval. No. 3 (National Bureau of Statistics), 1970, Table 54, pp.136–43.
2 Preston standard: see S. H. Preston, *Mortality Patterns in National Populations,* New York, Academic Press, 1976, Table 5.1, p. 91. The Preston standard is based on age-specific death rate data from Chile (4 dates), Taiwan (3 dates), England and Wales (3 dates), South African Coloureds (one date), US Non-Whites (one date) and Japan, 1993, itself.
3 Japan 1908: Values taken from S. H. Preston, N. Keyfitz and R. Schoen, *Causes of Death. Life Tables for National Populations,* New York, Seminar Press, 1972, pp. 420–2. The ratios are based on the death rates expressed as Mx values (population age-specific death rates) not the Qx values.

in India is even lower at 8 per cent. India was well known as an infanticidal culture, and the reduced survival advantage of female infants probably reflects that fact. But by comparing Japan to other countries, it begins to look as if there was some relative excess female mortality for Japanese infants, as if female infanticide was practised in Meiji Japan, as it is believed to have been earlier.[33]

If this is true, continuing female infanticide could not be blamed on the *explicit policies* of the Meiji government. Quite the contrary. The government was committed to encouraging rapid population growth, and the suppression of infanticide, male or female, was part of its population policy, as was preventing the diffusion of contraception, or knowledge about it. To enforce its demographic policies the state converted midwives into reproductive policewomen, who were sworn to prevent infanticide and report any suspicious infant deaths. In response, some Japanese women chose to give birth alone, rather than have well-trained midwives interfere with the degree of control they had over their own realised fertility.[34] Obviously this escape from trained midwives would place the lives of some adult women at risk, even though it permitted some sex selection to continue.

To understand why women might want to avoid raising a daughter (or another daughter) we would have to consider how other state policies made such a choice 'rational'. In general, as we shall see, the Meiji government adopted policies which made Japanese wives more, not less, dependent on their adult sons for old age support than they had ever been. A widow with no legitimate sons had no independent rights to land she had worked all her adult life. She and her legitimate daughters could be disinherited in favour of an illegitimate son, who could and would eject them from the family holding.[35]

Since there was no welfare system outside the family (and the resources generated by its land) the lot of the dispossessed widow was a sad and sorry one, as Japanese feminists noted.[36] By failing to give adult women independently assured property rights as wives (i.e. rights not derived through sons), the government implicitly encouraged female infanticide among peasant families, at the same time as it tried to prevent the destruction of infant life using midwives backed up by the rural police. The net effect of these inconsistent policies (if we assume that the infant mortality ratio should have been about 120, at the very least) was to implicitly encourage the deliberate elimination of about 8,000 female babies per year.[37]

If we assume that, nevertheless, some infant female lives were saved by government policy, we can ask what happened to them later. Female infants who were preserved against their parents' (or mother's) self-interested preferences might not have been cared for as carefully as more valued males. As a result, a kind of deferred infanticide seems to have emerged, in which some female babies who survived (because parents feared detection) died at a later stage due to relative neglect, thus causing the appearance of excess female mortality in early and later childhood (the age groups 1–4 years and 5–9 years).[38] This phenomenon – the replacement of outright infanticide with differential neglect – is thought to have occurred in India as a consequence of the anti-infanticide campaigns started under the British.

Using Preston's standard we can say that young Japanese girls were no worse off than was normal in low-life-expectancy, rural populations, but compared to Sweden they appear to be at a distinct disadvantage, especially in very early childhood (ages 1–4). Of the 63,168 girls aged 1–4 years who died in 1908, a few hundred might have been spared if we use Preston's standard. By Swedish standards many more should have survived, a few thousand more as 1–4 year olds, and another few thousand as 5–9 year olds. Picking a specific number depends on making an assumption about what the 'normal' or 'natural' mortality ratio should have been for the age groups in question.

DEVELOPMENT AND EXCESS FEMALE MORTALITY

It should not be imagined that the Meiji government had done nothing to improve the welfare of the young girls in its population. The reforming state made primary education compulsory for girls as well as boys, although in practice the quality of education received by girls was much lower. Classes for girls stressed the necessity of submitting to the authority of the state, fathers and husbands. After four to six years of this kind of 'education' many village girls were still functionally illiterate, but psychologically prepared to accept their relative powerlessness, and filled with a sense of strong obligation to repay their parents for the trouble of raising them.[39]

The government's campaigns to control epidemic disease, in particular those directed at eradicating smallpox, undoubtedly saved the lives of many boys and girls.[40] These campaigns may have added about four or five years to life expectancy at birth between 1870 and 1900.[41] But as life expectancy rose for both sexes, it rose more slowly for females. This pattern of differential improvement is similar to the demographic changes which took place in developing Western Europe.[42]

Even Sweden showed this pattern of slower improvement for girls,[43] so that while Swedish women 'started out' with a life expectancy at birth advantage of about four years over males (which they still had before the development process began) their advantage eroded to about two years after several decades of development, as female death rates failed to fall as fast as those of males in childhood and adolescence.

A similar process of change took place in South Asia, with females starting from a lower absolute advantage, and gradually developing a lower life expectancy at birth than that possessed by males.[44] A stylised version of the evolution of male/female life expectancy differences during development is presented in Figure 2.1.

In this diagram Japan is drawn as a middle line between the extreme of Northern Europe (based on the Swedish experience where excess female mortality was least pronounced) and South Asia, where it is most pronounced. But Japan's more remote

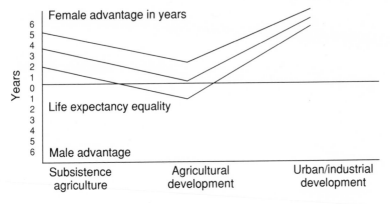

Figure 2.1 Life expectancy advantage at birth for males and females during development (in years)

Table 2.4 Life expectancy at birth: males and females, Japan, 1891–1975

Date	Males	Females	Difference
1891–9	42.8	44.3	1.5
1899–1903	44.0	44.9	0.9
1908	43.4	43.5	0.1
1909–13	44.3	44.7	0.4
1921–5	42.1	43.2	1.1
1926–30	45.0	46.5	1.5
1935–6	47.0	49.6	2.6
1947	50.1	54.0	3.9
1950–2	59.6	63.0	3.4
1955	63.6	67.8	4.2
1960	65.3	70.2	4.9
1965	67.7	73.0	5.3
1970	69.3	74.7	5.4
1975	71.1	77.0	5.3
1985	74.2	79.8	5.6

Source: The 14th Life Tables, Statistics and Information Department. Ministry of Health and Welfare, 1976.

history is hypothetical because reliable national data do not go back much before 1891–9. All we can see in the data available (see Table 2.4) is that females probably reached a nadir, in terms of their relative life expectancy advantage over males, in the first decade of the twentieth century.

Although no time series data exist for Japan as a whole,[45] the mortality history of the Hida area has been recovered from a Buddhist temple death register by Ann Jannetta and reconstructed jointly with Samuel Preston. Hida temple data show the predicted pattern.[46] The small mortality advantage of females declined over the nineteenth century, but Table 2.5 indicates that after four decades of development under Meiji policies female life expectancy at birth was four years lower than male life expectancy.

It is probably safe to say that even before the Meiji restoration, and its drive for development, the conditions under which Japanese women lived were not culturally advantageous. This is not surprising when we consider that Japan had been an officially patriarchal culture for centuries. But within that male-favouring framework historians and anthropologists agree that the status of women varied from era to era, place to place and class to class.[47]

Table 2.5 Male and female life expectancy at birth in a Hida
Prefecture Temple Death Register, various dates

Date	Male	Female	Difference
1776–95	32.5	33.6	1.1[1]
1856–75	29.2	29.8	0.6[1]
1876-95 [Meiji period]	38.9	36.0	–2.9[2]
1896–1915 [Meiji period]	38.9	34.8	–4.1[2]
1916–35	36.7	34.3	–2.4[2]
1936–55	37.1	39.1	2.0[1]

Notes: [1] = female advantage; [2] = male advantage

Source: Ann B. Janetta and Samuel Preston, 'Two Centuries of Mortality Change
in Central Japan: The Evidence from a Temple Death Register', *Population
Studies*, 1991, vol. 45, pp. 417–36.

Institutionalised patriarchal laws and customs fell with full force
only on upper-class women.

Despite regional variation in the status of women, pre-industrial
Japan may well have had its own 'missing women' problem. When
the total number of men counted in the Bakufu population surveys
of 1732 and l852 are divided by the number of women, very high
(male favouring) sex ratios are produced. (See Table 2.6.) By

Table 2.6 Sex ratios for selected countries in 1975 and Japan at
various dates (total male population over total female population)

Country	1732	1852	1908	1940	1975	
Japan	115	108	102	100	97	
England					95	(United Kingdom)
France					96	
Canada					100	
Mexico					102	
India					108	(Both countries exhibit pronounced excess female mortality)
Pakistan					114	

Sources: All values for 1975 are from the *United Nations Demographic Yearbook*
(1977), pp. 166–201. Values for Japan in 1732 and 1852 are from Irene Taeuber
(1958) based on Bakufu population counts of the village populations. *The
Population of Japan*, Princeton, Princeton University Press. Values from 1908
and 1940 are from Japanese census data.

twentieth-century standards eighteenth-century Japan looks like a society prone to female infanticide.[48]

But the Bakufu surveys had numerous defects. Some areas left out child populations altogether;[49] and only those individuals registered as belonging to specific households on a specific date were counted. Some itinerant workers were excluded as was the entire ruling class. If more itinerant workers were female than male, or polygyny was very extensive among feudal lords, then some living females might have not been counted. But the interpretation of this early data remains problematic.

Whatever the cause, by 1850 the reported sex ratio had dropped to 108,[50] and by 1908 it was 102, meaning that there was only a 2 per cent excess of males in the total population. At this time, however, some adult men were not in Japan itself, because of military service. Others had emigrated. Thus the almost equal numbers of men and women are misleading. This demonstrates that estimating how many females are 'missing' by looking at census sex ratios alone can underestimate the extent of excess female mortality, just as it fails to identify what stages of the life course are most differentially destructive of human life.[51]

Long run trends in Japan as a whole seem uncertain. Despite continuing controversy over how well or badly ordinary women fared before the Meiji restoration, widespread agreement seems to exist that the condition of women deteriorated afterwards, if not before.[52] During the entire Meiji restoration (1868–1912) as well as the subsequent Taisho (1912–26) era, the 'status' of women remained 'low', judged by the absence of legal and political rights, as well as the presence of excess female mortality. It was only after 1930, when male death rates rose to equal female rates, that sex-specific mortality ratios became less unequal. This new trend was related to the state's military policies,[53] as well as increasingly stressful conditions in the countryside.[54]

One thing seems fairly clear. The Meiji government succeeded in reducing regional and class-related variations in the position of women, thus creating a fairly standardised status pattern for women.[55] In theory, for example, before the Meiji restoration all women could be quickly and easily divorced by their husbands for any reason. In practice regional customs varied and, in any case, easy and frequent divorce may have worked for, not against, the ordinary peasant woman, especially given the apparent shortage of adult women in many Tokugawa villages.[56]

After the Meiji restoration the government began to discourage divorce, and divorced women began to suffer from a stigma which previously affected only upper-class women. In practice divorce remained easy for husbands, but wives could be 'sent away' for any minor reason – suspected adultery, or the failure to bear a male child. In theory a Japanese woman could also divorce her husband for adultery, but only after he had been found guilty in a court of law.[57]

While a marriage continued, a husband had the right to control any property or wages earned by his wife.[58] Adult women who married (and almost all did) had no control over or claim to the household's material resources, except that granted by a husband. The Meiji civil code of 1898 made the household into a micro institution whose male head was declared to be the official representative of the state in the lives of the household's members, wives, children and other relatives.[59] Every member of the household (the *ie*) was dependent on its resources, but it was the head who determined how and to what extent each person would share in those resources, as well as to what extent each member was expected to contribute. Since women could not become household heads they had no personal autonomy in the allocation of resources.[60] Women could only head households as an interim measure until a suitable male could be found by local authorities. Marriage became the only choice an adult women had, but that choice was not really hers to make. A marriage not approved by the male head of a woman's natal household would jeopardise a woman's claim to return and receive support if divorced. Since there were no social institutions designed to help the poor or distressed independently of the family (the absence of state-operated welfare-related institutions was the result of government policy), women became completely dependent on the will of a male household head. In general, men had rights and women had duties.

As the pre-war feminist Waka Yamada noted, when a household father protected and solicitously looked after his dependants, the loss of property rights did not matter. Loyalty and obedience were exchanged for protection and security. But that was the theory of the Meiji household. In practice, said Yamada, the position of women under Meiji law was a sorry spectacle. Husbands had authority without solicitude.[61] Marriage meant loss of autonomy, property rights, and a position of extreme dependence, in which a wife had to please, not only a new husband, but his mother, father and other relatives as well. If divorce occurred the only recourse for the rejected woman was to return to her natal family (without her children, over whom she had no legal rights), to a father or married brother who did not really want her back. Generally, women who did not achieve domestic security met a grim fate.[62] The lack of alternative opportunities meant that the status of a young wife was precarious and painful, even in the best of circumstances.

Given this situation it is not surprising that 33 per cent more women aged 25–29 died than men of the same age. Japanese women had an average age of marriage of around 23. After marriage the new wife was under extreme stress. Entering a household as an outsider who had to prove herself, she was expected to work twelve to thirteen hours a day, while trying to produce a viable male child to protect her own interests.

As long as fertility stayed high the state was indifferent to the welfare of young wives. It valued young women primarily as mothers, particularly of soldiers who would fight to expand Japan's empire.[63] It was their value to the state as mothers, which justified the suppression of reproductive autonomy in any form – infanticide, abortion or contraception. Although many women would have benefited from information on how to space births, the state outlawed the production and distribution of any kind of birth control information. The general impact of the state's policies was to leave rural women of reproductive age with as little control over their bodies as they had over any other form of property.

At any rate Japanese statistics for 1908 indicate that women in their late 20s and 30s (virtually all of them married) died at considerably higher rates than men from tuberculosis, as well as influenza, pneumonia, bronchitis and diarrhoea. Women also died at higher rates from chronic diseases like those afflicting the cardiovascular system, and cancer. Less than 7 per cent of these young women, dying in the age range 25–29, were victims of maternal mortality, which meant that death in childbirth (that is, at or near the time of childbirth) was a comparatively minor problem compared with death from infectious disease during the childbearing years. The greater susceptibility of women to disease, no doubt compounded by the stresses of pregnancy and childbirth, meant that 25–30 per cent more young women died than men. Had men and women died in approximately equal numbers during the age range 25–39 years (as in the Preston standard) at least 10,000 more young adult women would have lived longer than they did, on an annual basis.

No doubt poverty compromised the ability of young women to resist disease, or recover from its effects, but their excess mortality could also be a reflection of differential medical care. About one-third of all young women's deaths were classified as other and unknown (mostly the latter) during this period, while only one fourth of same age male deaths fell into this residual category.[64] 'Other and unknown' can be taken as an indicator of how many deaths took place without the attention of a Western-trained physician, who could provide the kind of diagnosis that led to a properly identified death. It is possible, then, that young adult women received less care during critical illnesses, especially since attention from a physician was relatively expensive. This supposition is strengthened by the fact that the statistical discrepancy between the sexes with respect to how deaths are classified, disappears abruptly once women reach the age of 45 years.

Japanese rural sociologists agree that upon reaching middle age Japanese rural women began to live much easier lives. As they became mothers of older children, or, best of all, mothers-in-law, their work loads lessened, their status rose, and their informal authority with respect to the household's resources increased. As mothers-in-law they were expected to do only light work, while allocating for themselves the best food, or whatever other privileges the household had to offer.[65] For older Japanese women life could be relatively pleasant; but of those females born after 1868 only about half could expect to live to 50 years of age. Subsequently that lucky (or hardy) half began to out-survive same age males; and they no longer died at higher rates from infectious and chronic disease, just as the percentage of deaths classified as 'other and unknown', dropped to approximately the same level as men's. Perhaps older Japanese women used their improved status to insist on more expensive or more extensive medical care than they could have obtained when younger.

Whatever the case, the state may have had no direct use for older women, but neither did it have any reason to make their lives worse. During the Meiji restoration the government continued to encourage respect for aged parents, including aged mothers, relying on the household to support the aged, thus

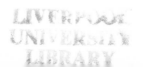

excusing the state from the expensive business of providing pensions in some form. Perhaps the prospect of old age security made women less resistant to overall government policy, and more willing to keep younger women in line.

In other words it would seem as if excess female mortality in Japan was an almost perfect reflection of the relative status of women within the household, in particular of the relative degree of control they had over material resources, as well as their own bodies. Nowhere is this more apparent than in the last age group to be considered here – young teens aged 10–14. As Table 2.1 shows, they also died at rates higher than those for same age males by about 33 per cent.

Developing Japan was a country short of capital whose major resource was its increasingly abundant labour supply. The Japanese government explicitly decided that one of the best ways to earn foreign currency was to combine the latest technology in silk and cotton textile manufacturing with the lowest cost, least-demanding workers – i.e. young female operatives. Not only were young girls educated for docility, but they expected to leave work upon marriage, which would make it difficult to unionise them. By minimising labour disputes, and using cheap labour, profits could be kept at a maximum, and so could taxes.

Thus 80 per cent of the workers in Japan's early twentieth-century textile factories were unmarried girls between the ages of 10 and 20 years, most of whom came from rural areas. To get them out of remote villages and into factories the government permitted labour recruiters to offer money to interested fathers in exchange for a daughter's labour. The contracts permitted girls as young as 10 years to be taken from their villages for a period of two or more years. These were renewable until the girl married or reached 21 years.[66] Until that time a girl's wages belonged to her household head, who had to pay a fee to the labour recruiter for arranging the job.

Thus the Japanese government socially constructed a labour market which made young girls into the prime source of indus-trial labour, and into a potential household asset for economically stressed households, and did this by imposing a kind of tempo-rary slavery on them. The girls, once contracted out, were forced to walk dozens or even hundreds of miles to their new place of employment, where they were housed in crowded dormitories and surrounded by high fences designed to prevent escape. Factory girls were fed regularly, but by all reports their diet was inadequate, given their long and arduous days. Discipline was severe, and sexual harassment routine.

It is no wonder that the first studies of factory workers showed that the girls who worked in them had death rates which were two to three times as high as those normal for their age group.[67] The government's own statistics were enough to shock reformers into action. They demanded that conditions in the factories be improved so as to save the 5,000 lives that Dr Osamu Ishirara estimated were sacrificed annually to keep Japan's textile industries highly profitable for owners and the government.[68]

Large numbers of older girls and young women were also employed in small-scale weaving shops. These household factories were equally exploitative, and unhealthy places to work. Worse still, many young girls were sold (again by their fathers) to brothels, where they eventually contracted one or more forms of venereal disease.[69] Given labour conditions, it is not surprising that thousands of adolescents and women ranging in age from 10 to 24 died premature deaths caused by a wide range of infectious diseases, but especially by tuberculosis. As textile workers, weavers or prostitutes, few girls had any real control over the kind of work they would do, or the conditions under which they would work. Had they died in numbers equal to those of males in this age range as many as 20,000 fewer premature deaths would have taken place each year, judging by the Preston standard.

In the final section we shall consider how Japan's policies with respect to women were selected in order to help Japan become a rich country with a strong army in as short a time as possible. This question is important because in the annals of world development Japan stands out as one of the best examples of a comprehensively planned approach to development,[70] based on the reconstruction of all its traditional political and social institutions. As a general rule the Japanese tried to import the latest and best from the West, whether that involved weapons or public health, industrial technology or medicine. But with respect to the household and women's status the Meiji reformers seemed determined *not to import* the latest social and institutional innovations, since they all involved improving the status of women. Instead of catching up with the West, the government officially extolled the glory of Japan's Confucian past, which had long insisted on the submission of women to their husbands.[71]

The government's policies towards the status of women were deliberately backward-looking, possibly because Japanese men were too selfish to give their own women more rights, and too willing to use the state to enforce their self-serving preferences. But it is also possible that the government's policies towards women were intended, like all the other policies, to promote development, strengthen the military, and permit imperial expansion. It is true that the submissive wife was an old Confucian ideal, but the Meiji government wanted women to be the devoted mothers of large families, as well as submissive wives (*ryosai kenbo*). In addition the government wanted submissive daughters who would work tirelessly and cheaply, withdrawing from the labour force at a suitable age.[72]

Such goals had no roots in Japan's Confucian past. Thus some social historians, after carefully considering the sources of Meiji government policy with respect to women, have concluded that the reformers were not drawing on Japan's remote past; they were drawing on Britain's relatively recent past.[73]

In effect, Japan's reformers were trying to import mid-Victorian England as the model for how to manage women during development. Victorian women were ceaselessly encouraged to submit to male authority. They had no property rights. Divorce was discouraged, but men could divorce their wives more easily than wives could divorce their husbands. (Japan's divorce law was almost identical to England's Matrimonial Causes Act of 1857.) The economic dependence of wives was held up as an ideal at the same time as many young British girls worked in textile factories during industrialisation. British women were excluded from political life as completely as Japanese women were after the peace preservation law of 1889 forbade women to join political associations, or attend political meetings.

Japanese officials may have believed that these restrictive laws would make marriages more stable, fertility higher and households richer, than would be the case under more liberal family policies. To Japanese eyes it must have seemed that early and mid-Victorian England had pioneered the successful management of women and families during development, despite the fact that the British government had no official policies with respect to these matters, any more than it had ever planned industrialisation.

But when late-nineteenth-century Japanese reformers observed developments in late-nineteenth-century England, what they saw was women demanding more rights, fertility declining, labour unrest increasing and the empire under attack. To Japanese officials feminism, unionism, declining birth rates and political dissent were all manifestations of individualism, which was considered the supreme threat to the state's drive for wealth and power. If Japan were to become a rich country with a strong army, as well as an expanding empire, both men and women would have to make sacrifices for the sake of the nation, not try to pursue their selfish interests during a time of rapid change.

Thus Japan's late-nineteenth-century government simply did not want to import the demographic and social consequences they thought of as associated with individualism, particularly rights for women. Ever watchful, the government eventually suppressed the publication of feminist literary magazines which glorified the value of romantic love, because marriages based on love were perceived as another manifestation of individualism, which challenged the legitimacy of marriages arranged for the sake of the household, and thus for the sake of the nation.

From the feminist perspective romantic love was part of the right to choose a husband, the hope being that within an affectionate marriage, wives would automatically have a better bargaining position. As it was, all Japanese feminists were permitted to do was advocate reforms designed to improve the welfare of mothers and children, or conditions in factories, because these measures were consistent with encouraging the growth of a healthy population.

By 1908 the Japanese government had every reason to suppose its harsh policies were working. Japan's population increased from about 35 million in the 1870s to 50 million by 1910.[74] Official statistics seemed to show that the birth rate continued to rise until 1920, about fifty years after it had begun to decline in Britain and Western Europe. If some women lost their lives in this great drive for national wealth and power, that was to be expected. As soldiers, ordinary men were also being asked to risk their lives for the sake of the state as soldiers in a series of wars.

Nevertheless, when we look at the statistics on male and female mortality ratios, it seems as if more women gave their lives for the nation more frequently, and at much younger ages than did men (at least until the 1930s). If we ask how many women may have lost their lives 'prematurely', in pursuit of the government's strategy for development, that remains a difficult question to answer. Had fewer females died as infants, children, teenagers and young mothers, how many would have survived to old age?

Let us make the very reasonable assumption that under less oppressive policies, the crude death rate for Japanese women could have been just one per thousand lower than it was for men in 1908. At that time the male crude death rate was 20.7 per thousand. If the female death rate had been just 19.7 per thousand (instead of 20.9 per thousand) 29,687 fewer Japanese females would have died that year. This is a very conservative estimate of annual excess female mortality, but it implies an avoidable loss of about 100,000 female lives every three to four years, with about 250,000 premature deaths in the first decade of the twentieth century alone.

Because the Japanese may have used mid-Victorian England as a guide to social policy during development, it is worth while comparing Japan's mortality ratios to those of England in the mid-Victorian period. In Table 2.7 we can see some striking similarities between the two patterns, along with some intriguing differences.

Like Japan, mid-Victorian England and Wales also had a form of excess female mortality in 1838–54. From the ages of 10 to 39 English and Welsh females died at higher rates than males, although not to the extent observed in Japan. But comparisons at the national level are somewhat misleading – England and Wales had the world's first urbanised population. Over half the population lived in cities, which meant that at mid-century the population was divided into two very different sectors; Japan, in contrast, was no more than 10 per cent urbanised in 1908, and most of its households still owned or rented land.

As can be observed, mortality ratios in the two sectors of mid-Victorian England were strikingly different, but neither rural nor urban England and Wales showed any sign of excess female mortality in infancy, possibly because the government had targeted infanticide for suppression as early as the 1600s. Moreover, the working-class women of England no longer gained access to landed property through married sons. Most families did not own or rent land, and so there was less socially constructed pressure on ordinary mothers to produce more sons than daughters to ensure their own old age security. Nevertheless rural England had a very pronounced form of excess female mortality, extending from the age of 5 to the age of 64 – in other words over a more extended part of the life span than in Japan. Why?

Table 2.7 Excess female mortality in Victorian England and Meiji Japan based on male/female age-specific mortality ratios (M/F)

Age group	England/Wales 1838–54	Rural England 1851–60†	Japan*
0–1	122	124	112
1–4	102	103	96
5–9	102	97	92
10–14	96	78	67
15–19	94	64	74
20–24	95	81	73
25–29	95	74‡	67
30–34	94	74	74
35–39	98	80‡	79
40–44	103	80	95
45–49	111	96‡	113
50–54	120	96	126
55–59	114	82‡	129
60–64	111	82	131
65–69	110	106‡	114
70–74	109	106	107
Life expectancy at birth	M=40; F=42	M=47; F=47	M=43; F=43

Notes:
* Japan was approximately 10% urban in 1908. Approximately 70% of the labour force was in the primary sector. England/Wales was about half rural at this period, with a substantial rural/industrial sector.
† = In 1851–60 life expectancy at birth for urban males was 33; for females it was 36 years.
‡ = Mortality ratio is given for a ten-year age group.
Sources: 1838–54 from W. Farr, *English Life Tables* (London, 1864); Rural England and Japan 1908: S. Preston, N. Keyfitz and R. Schoen, *Causes of Death. Life Tables for National Populations* (New York, 1976). G. Kearns (1993), 'Le Handicap Urbain et le Déclin de la Mortalité en Angleterre et au Pays de Galles 1851–1900', *Annales de Démographie Historique*, 75–105, see p. 93.

When historians describe the Victorian countryside during development, it is usually in terms which make ordinary women seem increasingly economically marginal during development.[75] The rural population of England was already wage-dependent before the industrial revolution began in the late eighteenth century. The enclosure movement combined with technological change gradually reduced the extent of employment in the agrarian sector of the economy. As jobs became scarce, males were given preference, and females found it harder and harder to earn money while remaining in the countryside.[76] Daughters who remained at home while unemployed were seen as increasingly burdensome to wage-dependent families. Their loss of relative economic value alone may account for the emergence of excess female mortality among the young, as ordinary rural English parents had to consider the relative merits of continuing to invest in the health or survival of sons versus daughters, just as their Indian counterparts are said to do in the twentieth century.

But the Japanese situation was very different. There, industrialisation was making young girls more, not less, potentially valuable to their families, albeit only if their fathers were willing to place their lives at risk in order to collect the wage attached to a job.

The common thread which joins two seemingly different situations is that whether or not young girls were becoming financial liabilities or assets to their families during development; they had no control over their lives in cultures which both devalued them and subsequently gave them little or no legal protection from either familial neglect or labour market exploitation. Whether or not employment opportunities decreased or increased, girls were deprived of the right to control resources, including their own bodies. Unless the state intervened to offer them special or compensatory forms of legal protection, at home or at work, some would die at an early age when subjected to biologically stressful conditions.

But mid-Victorian England offered a potential escape from rural powerlessness. More jobs were available for young English girls in cities, and in urban labour markets they seemed to have much more relative freedom, including the freedom to keep their own wages. Young women were reputed to be quick to leave one situation for another, if it seemed more advantageous to do so. Conservative Victorian moralists often claimed that urbanisation gave ordinary working girls too much freedom from family control, and/or too much bargaining power within the family.[77] Whatever the case there was no absolute excess female mortality in Victorian cities, despite the unhealthy disease environments which elevated the death rates of both sexes.[78]

But in Meiji Japan, as feminists noted, there was no place to hide from the government's family policies. Continual effort was exerted to see that young females would live and work under the same kind of oppressive patriarchal control everywhere.

Once married, Japanese women worked long and hard on the family farm. Landless rural wives in mid-nineteenth-century England did not have that option, and those who could not find paid work were extremely dependent on their wage-earning husbands. This total economic dependence is thought to have made it necessary for the wives of English labourers to stint themselves in order to feed their husbands. Given the prevalence of tuberculosis in mid-Victorian England, combined with the physiological demands imposed by pregnancy, it becomes easy to understand why so many more mid-Victorian rural women died of tuberculosis in the prime of their rural lives, although not necessarily of other diseases.[79]

In the end, what seems to matter most to the differential survival of males and females is not work or unemployment, but how labour markets are embedded in social systems which differentially value males and females, and thus differentially allocate the right to obtain and control resources. When female lives are devalued, this lesser value gets translated into a set of social conventions and explicit laws which restrict the positive rights of women, meaning their rights to control resources and invest those resources in their own welfare.

The most fundamental right to property is the ownership of one's own body. Without that all is slavery, irrespective of whether or not that word is used. The privileges associated with gender may have their roots in tradition, but most rights to own and control resources (including one's body) become the subject of intense consideration during development. Similarly, policy issues involving relative welfare come to the fore, as societies decide who will gain most or lose most during a period of rapid change.

In developing Japan it was explicitly decided by all-male governments that development would mean that ordinary men had new rights while ordinary women had new duties. In developing Britain informal political and social policies, also dominated by men, had come to the same conclusion without making explicit policy decisions. The best thing the British government did for ordinary women was to adopt a kind of benign neglect towards the urban working-class family and their female members, which meant that patriarchal norms and behaviours were not policed as stringently as they were in Japan.

The most striking contrast between the mortality ratios of mid-Victorian England and Meiji Japan are found among older women. As we have seen, older women in Japan did quite well after they reached middle age. In England those rural women who lived past 50 years did not live longer than men of the same age. Since married children in England did not normally live with their adult parents, maturity did not involve any sort of promotion to a privileged status. In general, old age meant increasing poverty and sometimes greater isolation for both men and women. Although the English poor law ensured that every impoverished person would get some kind of parochial assistance, poor rural women may have been fairly debilitated after a life-time of sacrifice, and public support did not mean a secure or pleasant old age.

In both countries the state's officials were aware that excess female mortality existed. The British government did not regard it as a major social problem, and nothing was ever done about it. As the urban sector expanded, excess female mortality disappeared from the national statistics. In Japan, excess female mortality was regarded as a problem only insofar as it affected textile workers. A few reforms were undertaken to improve their condition after 1910. But in both countries the female lives lost prematurely were not perceived as a threat to the country, as long as high fertility continued to fuel rapid population growth.

It remains tempting to believe that if developing Japan or rural Victorian England had had higher per capita incomes, they would have had less excess female mortality. While this cannot be disproved, it is salutary to note that excess female mortality existed in the United States as well, despite its income advantages.[80] In the 1880s, when such families had per capita incomes five to ten times greater than those of Japanese peasants, girls aged 10–19 nevertheless died at rates 10–20 per cent higher than those of boys.

American historians who have looked at the data often stress that from the standpoint of excess female mortality, things seemed worse for 'upper-wealth-class' rural girls than for those who came from less well-off families.[81] Girls from landowning families in the United States also suffered from a legal system which made it difficult to own and control property, just as they found it difficult to obtain paid employment outside the home. In mid-Victorian England excess female mortality did not exist among urbanised populations in general, but it did exist among propertied middle-class families who lived in cities.[82] For a time, it even existed in Britain's aristocracy.

The aristocratic cohorts characterised by excess female mortality in Britain consisted of those females born in the first half of the eighteenth century. Dowries were exceptionally high at the time, and the marriage prospects of inadequately endowed daughters were uncertain. Despite their seemingly privileged circumstances, 'surplus' daughters were regarded as costly and socially problematic. We know that they died young at higher rates than the boys belonging to these wealthy families from the very first year of life through to the age of 10 years. As economically privileged women they also continued to die at higher rates during the childbearing years and, surprisingly, right on through late middle age to the age of 59 years.[83]

During this period of excess female mortality among the very rich, the rights of married women to exercise control over any form of property after marriage were being steadily eroded in courts of law.[84] As the legal historian Susan Staves explains, the increasingly male-favouring property regime of eighteenth-century England was only made possible by support from a male-dominated state, which was ideologically biased against any form of economic independence for women. Upper-class women were seen as little more than procreators, not as individuals in need of equal legal rights. (This, of course, was the same philosophy adopted by the government of Meiji Japan.)

Privileges without rights do not necessarily translate into lives that are happy, healthy or long. Perhaps that is one reason upper- and middle-class women in England and the United States gave so much support to the idea of romantic love, hoping (like their Japanese counterparts in the early twentieth century) that affection could get them better treatment within marriage than the law was prepared to offer.

In short, those modern demographers who argue that excess female mortality will not disappear in their countries until the state strengthens the rights of women, young and old, are being more than politically correct.[85] They are, in all probability, demographically correct.

Excess female mortality disappeared in Japan after World War II. It is true that this disappearance must have been assisted by the end of the drive for military expansion, and the resumption of economic growth, but the old household system and the laws which maintained it were also abolished in response to American pressure.

The post-war reforms conferred a legal and social identity on women, independent of membership in a household ruled autocratically by a male head. The laws which forbade abortion were also repealed. Fertility fell rapidly after 1950, a fact which must have reduced the production of unwanted daughters. Although Japanese women are still a long way from genuine social equality with males, they have the kind of formal equality which confers on them the rights to produce and control resources necessary for the protection of health, including the right to manage their own body for reproductive purposes.

NOTES

1 Delivered at the conference on Gender, Health and Welfare at Oxford Brooks University, 6 November 1993; revised for British Society for Population Studies Meeting: Gender, Demography and the Social Structure of Japan in the Past, at the Cambridge Group for the History of Population and Social Structure, Cambridge University, 3 March 1994. Delivered at St Antony's College, Oxford, 27 May 1994. The author wishes to thank Anne Digby, Richard Smith, Ann Waswo, Richard Wall, Laurel Cornell and Saito Osamu for their comments on earlier drafts. All responsibility for errors and oversimplifications remains mine.

2 Estimates of missing women are based on a comparison of expected versus observed sex ratios as reported in national censuses. Sex ratios are calculated as the total number of enumerated men divided by the total number of enumerated women.

3 See Amartya Sen, 'Missing Women', *British Medical Journal*, 7 March 1992, pp. 587–8. See also Sen's article in the *New York Review of Books*, 'More than 100 Million Women are Missing', 20 December 1990, pp. 61–6. Sen's 'missing women' estimates are based on assumptions about what sex ratios are normal for large populations which are censused, given a certain level of life expectancy.

   Ansley Coale disputed the methods used by Sen to estimate the number of missing women. See Coale, 'Excess Female Mortality and the Balance of the Sexes', *Population and Development Review*, 1991, vol. 17, pp. 517–23. Stephen Klasen compared and evaluated the range of methods used by both Sen and Coale, and to re-estimate the number of missing women based on sex ratios using still other assumptions about what is normal, in ' "Missing Women" Reconsidered', forthcoming, *World Development*.

4 S. Ryan Johansson, 'Welfare, Mortality and Gender: Continuity and Change in Theories About Male/Female Mortality Differentials Over Three Centuries', *Continuity and Change*, 1991, vol. 6, pp. 135–77.

5 Jane Humphries, ' "Bread and a Pennyworth of Treacle": Excess Female Mortality in England in the 1840s', *Cambridge Journal of Economics*, 1991, vol. 15, pp. 451–73.

6 Dean Gerstein, R. Duncan Luce, Neil J. Smelser and Sonja Sperlich

(eds), *The Behavioural and Social Sciences*, Washington D.C., National Academy Press, 1988, p. 135.

7 Edward Shorter, *A History of Women's Bodies*, New York, Basic Books, 1991. Shorter explained the existence of excess female mortality by arguing that in the past, before the advent of fertility control and modern health care, women were inherently less healthy than men, and therefore died at higher rates than men. But Shorter assumed that excess female mortality had always characterised the demography of rural areas. In fact extensive excess female mortality was a relatively new phenomenon which emerged during the early stages of economic development in rural areas, and disappeared with increasing urbanisation. For a detailed critique of Shorter's treatment of excess female mortality, see S. Ryan Johansson, 'Women's Bodies: A Review Essay', *Historical Methods*, 1984, vol. 17, pp. 33–7.

8 M. Rosenzweig and T. P. Schultz, 'Market Opportunities, Genetic Endowment and Intra-Family Resource Distribution', *American Economic Review*, 1982, vol. 72, pp. 803–15.

9 Sonalde Desai and Devaki Jain, 'Maternal Employment and Changes in Family Dynamics: the Social Context of Women's Work in Rural South India', *Population and Development Review*, 1994, vol. 20, pp. 115–36.

10 UNICEF's publication called *The Girl Child: An Investment in the Future* describes the unfavourable position of young girls in developing countries using a range of economic statistics but explains inferior treatment in terms of prejudices 'rooted in culture and customs', New York, 1990, p. 14.

11 Alaka M. Basu, *Culture, the Status of Women and Demographic Behavior: Illustrated with the Case of India*, Oxford, Clarendon Press, 1992.

12 For a review of the historical data for India and Sri Lanka (formerly Ceylon) Christopher Langford and Pamela Story, 'Sex Differentials in Mortality Early in the Twentieth Century: Sri Lanka and India Compared', *Population and Development Review*, 1993, vol. 9, pp. 263–81.

13 Barbara Miller, *The Endangered Sex: The Neglect of Female Children in Rural North India*, Ithaca, Cornell University Press, 1982.

14 For an argument that all market processes are socially embedded in a wider cultural contex see Mark Granovetter, 'Economic Action and Social Structure: A Theory of Embeddedness', *American Journal of Sociology*, 1985, vol. 91, pp. 481–510.

15 David Kertzer and Denis Hogan, *Family, Political Economy and Demographic Change*, Madison, University of Wisconsin Press, 1989. See also Barry Feldman, 'Networks, Externalities, Local Interaction and Some of the Missing Links Between Individual and Aggregate Behavior', paper presented at the Fifth International Conference of the Society for the Advancement of Socio-Economics, 26–28 March 1993.

16 Richard M. Titmuss, *Birth, Poverty and Wealth*, London, Hamish Hamilton Medical Books, 1943, p. 5.

17 David Reisman, *The Political Economy of Health Care*, New York, St Martin's Press, 1993.
18 Alan L. Mackay, *A Dictionary of Scientific Quotations*, Bristol, Institute of Physics Publishing, 1991, p. 171.
19 See Jean-Baptiste Say, *Traité d'économie politique*, 1803. The demographically focused passages of this treatise were excerpted and translated in *Population and Development Review*, 1993, vol. 19, pp. 349–63. Say recognised that the government could take human lives directly (through war and other organised forms of violence) or indirectly, for example through punitively high levels of taxation, p. 355.
20 Modern economics, in the form of neo-classical economics, more or less minimises the role played by the state in all patterned forms of human behaviour for both theoretical and methodological reasons. See K. W. Rothchild, 'The Neglect of Power in Economics', in K. W. Rothchild (ed.), *Power in Economics*, Harmondsworth, England, Penguin Books, 1971, pp. 20–4. See also E. Ronald Walker, 'Beyond the Market', in K. W. Rothchild (ed.), *Power in Economics*, Harmondsworth, England, Penguin Books, 1971, pp. 42–54. For a more recent treatment see Terence Hutchison, *Changing Aims in Economics*, Oxford, Blackwell, 1992.
21 Amartya Sen, 'The Economics of Life and Death', *Scientific American*, May 1993, pp. 18–25.
22 Harold Wilensky *et al.*, *Comparative Social Policy. Theories, Methods, Findings*, Institute of International Studies, Berkeley, University of California, 1985, p. 49.
23 Samuel Preston, *Mortality Patterns in National Populations*, New York, Academic Press, 1976. Preston's arguments have been disputed or ignored by scholars who uphold the superior value of rising incomes and better nutrition. For a review of the debate see S. Ryan Johansson, 'Food for Thought: Rhetoric and Reality in Modern Mortality History', *Historical Methods*, 1994, vol. 27, pp. 101–26.
24 Sonalde Desai and Devaki Jain, 'Maternal Employment and Changes in Family Dynamics: the Social Context of Women's Work in Rural South India', *Population and Development Review*, 1994, vol. 20, pp. 115–36. See also Kertzer and Hogan, *Family Political Economy and Demographic Change*, p. 185.
25 For an explanation of how implicit policy can drive a fertility transition without conscious intention on the part of the government, see S. Ryan Johansson, 'Implicit Policy and Fertility During Development', *Population and Development Review*, 1991, vol. 17, pp. 377–414.
26 W. W. Lockwood, *The Economic Development of Japan. Growth and Structural Change*, Princeton, Princeton University Press, 1954.
27 Nobuhiko Murakami, *Meiji Jyoseishi* (History of Women in the Meiji Era), Tokyo, Kabushikigaisha Rironsha, 1971.
28 Andrew Fraser, 'Local Administration: the Example of Awa-Tokushima', in Marius Jansen and G. Rozman (eds), *Japan in Transition: From Tokugawa to Meiji*, Princeton, Princeton University Press. On p. 112 Fraser shows that 40 per cent of locally raised tax

revenues went to fund the police force, versus 30 per cent for other administrative expenses combined, and 30 per cent for education, public works and other expenditures (combined).

29 Some aspects of family life were also policed in late nineteenth- and early twentieth-century Europe, but as Jacques Donzelot points out, the policing of families in Western Europe was generally designed to weaken certain patriarchal aspects of family life, not to strengthen them. See *The Policing of Families*, New York, Pantheon, 1979.

30 Ingrid Waldron, 'The Role of Genetic and Biological Factors in Sex Differences in Mortality', in A. Lopez and L. Ruzsicka (eds), *Sex Differences in Mortality*, Canberra, Australian National University, 1983, pp. 141–64.

31 Samuel Preston, *Mortality Patterns in National Populations*, New York, Academic Press, 1976. See p. 91.

32 Today a normal value for this ratio is 120 to 130. See Sten Johansson and Ola Nygren, 'The Missing Girls of China: A New Demographic Account', *Population and Development Review*, 1991, vol. 17, pp. 35–51.

33 For the debate over the extent of infanticide in eighteenth- and early nineteenth-century Japan see Osamu, Saito, 'Infanticide, Fertility and "Population Stagnation": The State of Tokugawa Historical Demography', *Japan Forum*, 1992, vol. 4, pp. 369–82.

34 Robert Smith and Ella Lury Wiswell, *The Women of Suya Mura*, Chicago, University of Chicago Press, 1982. Smith's book is based on field notes of Ella Wiswell who as Ella Embree lived in the village of Suya Mura with her husband in the 1930s. Wiswell spoke Japanese and received glimpses into women's private lives that her anthropologist husband was denied. It was Wiswell who reported the tendency of these poor rural women to give birth alone, rather than call in the midwife (p. 273).

35 Nobuiko Murakami, *Meiji Jyoseishi* (History of Women in the Meiji Era), Tokyo, Kabushikigaisha Rironsha, 1971.

36 Joyce Lebra, Joy Paulson and Elizabeth Powers, *Women in Changing Japan*, Boulder, Westview Press, 1976.

37 This estimate uses the 1908 data provided in S. Preston, N. Keyfitz and R. Schoen, *Causes of Death. Life Tables for National Populations*, New York, Seminar Press, 1972, pp. 420–2. It begins with the assumption that the mortality ratio for infant deaths (M/F) in 1908 should have been 120 at the very least, not 112.

38 S. Ryan Johansson, 'Deferred Infanticide: Excess Female Mortality in Childhood', in G. Hausfater and Sarah Hardy (eds), *Infanticide*, New York, Aldine, 1984, pp. 463–86.

39 N. Murakami, *Meiji Jyoseishi*, 1971, p. 10.

40 S. Ryan Johansson and Carl Mosk, 'Exposure, Resistance and Life Expectancy: Disease and Death During the Economic Development of Japan, 1900–1960', *Population Studies*, 1987, vol. 41, pp. 207–35.

41 Ann Bowman Janetta and Samuel Preston, 'Two Centuries of Mortality Change in Central Japan: The Evidence from a Temple Death Register', *Population Studies*, 1991, vol. 45, pp. 417–36.

42 Dominique Tabutin, 'La Surmortalité feminine en Europe avant 1940', *Population*, 1978, vol. 33, pp 121–48. Tabutin attributes the emergence of excess female mortality to capitalist industrialisation. But since excess female mortality was largely a rural phenomenon, this explanation seems inappropriate unless capitalist industrialisation includes the commercialisation of agriculture.

43 S. Ryan Johansson, 'Deferred Infanticide: Excess Female Mortality in Childhood', in G. Hausfater and Sarah Hardy (eds), *Infanticide*, New York, Aldine, 1984, pp. 463–86.

44 For a review of the historical data for India and Sri Lanka (formerly Ceylon), see Christopher Langford and Pamela Story, 'Sex Differentials in Mortality Early in the Twentieth Century: Sri Lanka and India Compared', *Population and Development Review*, 1993, vol. 19, pp. 263–81.

45 Akira Hayami, 'Population Changes', in M. Jansen and G. Rozman (eds), *Japan in Transition: From Tokugawa to Meiji*, Princeton, Princeton University Press, pp. 280–7.

46 Ann Bowman Janetta and Samuel Preston, 'Two Centuries of Mortality Change in Central Japan: The Evidence from a Temple Death Register', *Population Studies*, 1991, vol. 45, pp. 417–36.

47 Mariko Tamanoi, 'Women's Voices: Their Critique of the Anthropology of Japan', *Annual Review of Anthropology*, 1990, vol. 19, pp. 17–37.

48 Irene Taeuber, *The Population of Japan*, Princeton, Princeton University Press, 1958, pp. 21–2.

49 Akira Hayami, 'Population Changes', in Jansen and Rozman, *Japan in Transition*, pp. 280–7.

50 Hayami, 'Population Changes', p. 314.

51 It is possible that in the eighteenth century female infanticide was widespread in Japan, so that all unwanted girls were eliminated shortly after birth. This would account for the fact that so little excess female mortality shows up in the studies of individual villages from that period.

52 Joyce Lebra, Joy Paulson and Elizabeth Powers, *Women in Changing Japan*, Boulder, Westview Press, 1976.

53 Irene Taeuber, *The Population of Japan*, pp. 308–10.

54 T. Tango and S. Kurashina, 'Age, Period and Cohort Analysis of Trends in Mortality from Major Diseases in Japan 1955–1979: Peculiarity of the Cohort Born in the Early Showa Era', *Statistics in Medicine*, 1987, vol. 6, pp. 709–26. The early Showa Era cohorts were children in the 1930s.

55 James White, *The Demography of Sociopolitical Conflict in Japan 1721–1846*, Berkeley, Institute of East Asian Studies, University of California, 1992. Prior to the Meiji restoration the regions of Japan were still differentiated with respect to laws and customs.

56 Laurel Cornell, 'Peasant Women and Divorce in Pre-industrial Japan: was "Three-and-a-half Lines" so Bad?', *Signs*, 1990, vol. 15, p. 4.

57 Robert J. Smith, 'Gender Inequality in Contemporary Japan', *Journal of Japanese Studies*, 1987, vol. 13. p. 9.

58 Ibid., p. 9.
59 Harold Wilensky, *The Welfare State and Equality*, Tokyo, Bokutakusha Publishing Co., 1984, pp. 2–14.
60 Nobuhiko Murakami, *Meiji Jyoseishi* (History of Women in the Meiji Era), Tokyo, Kabushikigaisha Rironsha, 1971.
61 Waka Yamada, *The Social Status of Japanese Women*, Tokyo, Kokusai Bunka Shinkokai, 1937. For a feminist critique of the position of women from 1868 to 1940 see S. Seiver, *Flowers in Salt: the Beginnings of Feminist Consciousness in Japan*, Stanford, Stanford University Press, 1983.
62 Robert J. Smith, op. cit., p. 13.
63 N. Murakami, *Meiji Jyoseishi* (History of Women in the Meiji Era), 1971.
64 S. Preston, N. Keyfitz and R. Schoen, *Causes of Death. Life Tables for National Populations*, New York, Seminar Press, 1972, pp. 420–2.
65 Richard K. Beardsly, *Village Japan*, Chicago, University of Chicago Press, 1959.
66 E. Patricia Tsurmi, *Factory Girls*, Princeton, Princeton University Press, 1990.
67 Margaret Powell and Masahira Amesaki, *Medical Care in Japan*, London, Routledge, 1990, p. 45. In 1888, 92 per cent of those prostitutes checked by physicians had one or more forms of venereal disease.
68 Ibid., p. 45.
69 Ibid., p. 39. These data come from physicians who examined a sample of prostitutes.
70 Jean-Jaques Salomon and Andre Lebeau, *Mirages of Development*, London, Lynne Rienner Publishers, 1993; W. W. Lockwood, *The Economic Development of Japan: Growth and Structural Change*, Princeton, Princeton University Press, 1954.
71 Joyce Lebra, Joy Paulson and Elizabeth Powers, *Women in Changing Japan*, Boulder, Westview Press, 1976.
72 Robert J. Smith, 'Making Village Women Into "Good Wives and Wise Mothers" in Prewar Japan', *Journal of Family History*, 1983, vol. 8, pp. 70–94; S. Koyma, 'Ryosai Kenbo Shugi No Reimei', *Josei-gaku Nempo*, 1986, vol. 7, pp. 11–20.
73 Ibid., and S. H. Nolte, 'Women The State and Repression in Imperial Japan', Michigan State University, Working Paper, Women in International Development, 1983.
74 Demographic Statistics 1986, Institute of Population Problems, Ministry of Health and Welfare, Tokyo, 1986.
75 Keith Snell, *Annals of the Labouring Poor*, Cambridge, Cambridge University Press, 1988.
76 Robert Allen, *Enclosure and the Yeoman*, Oxford, Clarendon Press, 1992, p. 287.
77 S. Ryan Johansson, 'Sex and Death in Victorian England', in Martha Vicinus (ed.), *Suffer and Be Still*, Bloomington, Indiana University Press, 1971, pp. 163–81.
78 Jane Humphries, ' "Bread and a Pennyworth of Treacle": Excess

Female Mortality in England in the 1840s', *Cambridge Journal of Economics*, 1991, vol. 15, pp. 451–73. Humphries finds some relative excess female mortality among middle-aged women living in cities.

79 Ibid. See also S. Ryan Johansson, 'Sex and Death in Victorian England', in Martha Vicinus (ed.), *Suffer and Be Still*, Bloomington, Indiana University Press, 1971, pp. 163–81.

80 For data on the excess female mortality in the United States in the late nineteenth century see G. Condran and E. Crimmons, 'A Description and Evaluation of the Mortality Data in Federal Censuses: 1850–1900', *Historical Methods*, 1979, vol. 12, pp. 1–15. See especially p. 12. For data from Massachusetts see C. Ginsberg and A. Swedlund, 'Sex-specific Mortality and Economic Opportunity: Massachusetts, 1860–1899', *Continuity and Change*, 1986, vol. 1, pp. 415–46.

81 R. Meindl, 'Family Formation and Health in 19th Century Franklin County, Massachusetts', in B. Dyke and W. Morrill (eds), *Genealogical Demography*, New York, Academic Press, 1980, pp. 235–50.

82 Joseph Fox, 'On the vital statistics of the Society of Friends', *Journal of the Statistical Society of London*, June, 1859. See p. 220.

83 T. H. Hollingsworth, 'Mortality and the British Peerage', *Population*, 1977, *Numero Special*, pp. 323–52.

84 Susan Staves, *Married Women's Separate Property in England 1660–1833*, Cambridge, Cambridge University Press, 1990.

85 Zeng Yi, Tu Ping *et al.*, 'Causes and Implications of the Recent Increase in the Reported Sex Ratio at Birth in China', *Population and Development Review*, 1993, vol. 19, pp. 283–301. For a general treatment of the relationship between rights and life expectancy during development see Partha Dasgupta, 'Well-being, Foundations and Extent of its Realisation in Poor Countries', *Economic Journal*, 1990, vol. 100, supplement, pp. 1–32.

Chapter 3

Poverty, health, and the politics of gender in Britain 1870–1948[1]

Anne Digby

Attention has shifted in feminist work from the later to the earlier
stages of welfare and health systems. With this has come a rein-
terpretation, since some early welfare systems between the 1880s
and 1920s are now seen to have borne strongly maternalist char-
acteristics.[2] In focusing on earlier voluntarist phases of health and
welfare programmes, the significance of female voluntary and civic
groups is recognised as having been instrumental in the formation of state policies.[3] In the USA and in Italy policies focusing
on maternity emerged at the very beginning of welfare provision.
In the USA women had very early access to education, and female
energies were focused in secular women's organisations and were
not diverted into the voluntary bodies of a state church. Crucially
there was a political space for maternalist social policies because
of the absence of paternalist welfare provision in a 'weak' state.
In forty states between 1911 and 1920 unsupported mothers were
granted pensions (the so-called widow's pensions) as a result of
state-by-state efforts of largely women's organisations linked to a
media campaign.[4] In Italy, the National Maternity Fund of 1910
was the outcome of a successful women's movement that had
emphasised the claim of women to a female citizenship which was
rooted in their rôle as mothers, and to the rights of mothers.[5] In
Britain, and in many other countries, another model was adopted
and such policies were part of an interrelated complex of paternalist and maternalist reforming initiatives. In each model an
analysis of the role of early feminist and women's organisations
– that earlier had been relegated to footnote status in traditional
histories of the rise of welfare states – becomes central. In British
feminist historiography this new interest in maternalism is part of
a more general conceptual shift from a concentration on female

suffrage towards an appreciation of gendered citizenship, and of women's part in what has been termed municipal housekeeping. Rather than focusing only on gender domination and inequality, women's own social solidarity and moral purpose and their authority as mothers is highlighted in interpretations which emphasise separateness and difference in gender roles. Significantly, the boundaries of the state are also redrawn to extend beyond a narrow focus on central government to an analysis of a domestified politics in the community and the local state. However, Jane Lewis has referred to the 'slipperiness of the concept of maternalism' in that while historians who use the term always emphasise female agency, the location and aims of this agency show wide variation.[6]

This chapter explores the extent to which British welfare was maternalist by looking first at poverty and then at health. It focuses on women as providers, managers, consumers and in networks and asks whether women were able to implement Eleanor Rathbone's agenda for welfare feminism of 1925. She stated that:

> We can stop looking at all our problems through men's eyes and discussing them in men's phraseology. We can demand what we want for women, not because it is what men have got, but because it is what women need to fulfil the potentialities of their own natures and to adjust themselves to the circumstances of their own lives.[7]

The chapter also analyses the degree to which that agenda was distinct from that of equal rights feminists, in seeing women as mothers rather than as individuals in their own right. It ends by assessing the extent to which the classic welfare state of the 1940s thus implemented an earlier maternalist welfare agenda rather than a universalist one.

POVERTY

Among social policy commentators there has been a recent discovery of the so-called 'feminisation of poverty'. Yet historical studies of the poor law as far back as the seventeenth century have revealed that women were in the majority among recipients of welfare. At the time of a major enquiry into the poor laws in the 1900s, for example, women formed three-fifths of those on all forms of poor relief.[8] In practice they were therefore the major clients of the poor law, but the framers of the poor law always had the adult male worker at the centre of their policy considerations. Women were seen almost exclusively as dependants under the Victorian and Edwardian poor law.[9]

It is interesting to find, however, that the poor law as the central statutory welfare agency had not been totally repellent to Victorian wives in their role as consumers of welfare and thus as providers for their families. They were able to manipulate assistance from the poor law; not just in the form of medicines and food from the medical officer but also as monetary assistance from the guardians, so that poor relief could become a not insignificant element in household resources.[10] So while the stereotype of the female applicant is of powerlessness and passivity there was some potential for empowerment. Similarly, women's knowledge of varied charitable assistance meant that resources could be increased by good management. Economic survival for the working class might depend on knowledge by the mother of ways through and around the multitude of relief and charitable agencies, with children acting as their agents. A childhood recollection from a man born in 1886 illustrated this well:

> I've been to Uncle Sam's breakfast at half past eight. I've been to Shepherd Street Mission round the corner here at nine o'clock and I've been to some other organisations for my breakfast at ten o'clock. ... I've had my mother meeting me and taking them home while I've gone to the next place and then when I come out of the next place she met me and took them home until I've got as many as four on Christmas morning. Not only me but scores of kiddies used to do the same thing.[11]

Not that every working-class woman would wish to rely on charity to manage the household budget since financial independence was prized, and the intrusiveness of state and voluntary agencies viewed with suspicion and dislike by the respectable working class.[12] Take this statement by a woman born in 1913, 'In those days if you got money on the cheap ... well you lived on charity and the neighbours would let you know, they're living on charity, living on the town.'[13] Given these attitudes women's self-help was of obvious importance. This was not the masculine individual and privatised version championed earlier by Samuel Smiles but was collective, based on a gendered solidarity of mutuality, and centred on informal familial and neighbourly networks.[14] It is revealing to find Hannah Mitchell, one of the few early working-class women who held public office, later town councillor and member of the public assistance committee for Manchester, reviewing her time as a Poor Law Guardian for Ashton and deciding that her ability to do so was dependent on such networks. Without a good neighbour to cook the Mitchell family's midday dinner on the weekly committee day Hannah recognised that she would have been unable to perform her onerous public service in either town.[15]

The continued role of women as household managers is well illustrated by the hidden but vital work they did during the hard years of the inter-war depression. The tight squeeze on poor relief (later termed public assistance) given to families during the economically depressed inter-war period was notorious and certain areas of the country in Durham, South Wales and London led the political fight against it. Their stance was encapsulated in George Lansbury's words that, 'If people starve on wages, there is no reason why they should starve on relief.'[16] A clear idea of the difference of view about what was needed to run a household is given if we compare the figures on sums needed to run a household administered by elected guardians in the Durham union of Chester le Street with those given by centrally appointed guardians whom the central government later imposed upon them during the Coal Lock-Out of 1926. Within four months they had cut relief to the wives of those in dispute by two-fifths from 15, to 12 and then to 8 shillings a week, while child allowances were reduced from 5 to 2 shillings. Earlier, the ministry had considered 12 shillings and 4 shillings respectively were reasonable sums. The household relief scale with a maximum of 50 shillings was cut by 30 per cent and in applying it, *all* offsetting household resources were taken into account, from small capital in bank and savings books down to children's free school meals, or Co-op dividends.[17] In these circumstances there was contemporary concern over health and the National Birthday Trust's survey of maternal mortality in Durham and South Wales found mothers severely undernourished. It was this – rather than lack of medical care – that it concluded was the key factor in high maternal mortality rates.[18] While the experience of these Durham women was unusually difficult, all households dependent on relief or assistance came under pressure with the squeeze on public expenditure. Poor Law

Guardians (or their successors, the members of public assistance committees) also tried to extend familial responsibilities when hard-pressed ratepayers were protesting about the perceived burden of high poor rates.[19] There was thus a gap between law and practice, the latter being driven by economic considerations. The family as a convenient form of caring remained a useful substitute for more expensive institutional care. Here women were in the front-line as welfare providers in their roles as familial carers for the old and/or disabled, as well as for their husbands and children.

That this was the case was linked to the fact that only about one in ten married women were full-time workers or providers in the inter-war labour market. Restrictions on eligibility for welfare benefits of various kinds affected both men and women but, in addition, women faced some gender-specific discrimination within the unemployment insurance system of 1911. (See also the later chapter by Jane Lewis for a discussion of this.) It is illuminating to see that William Beveridge, writing in 1930, referred to 'claims by women who on marriage had practically retired from the industry and were not wanted by employers, but tried not unnaturally to get something for nothing out of the fund'. This was one of the few instances when he thought the 'genuinely seeking work' test of the period was not dishonourable but justified.[20] By the early 1930s there was anxiety among the Ministry of Health's officials about the 'symptoms of the beginnings or spread of social disease', by which was meant welfare dependency.[21] During the late 1920s and early 1930s there was concern about an 'increasing tendency to seek for public assistance of some kind in time of stress',[22] so that 'the old reluctance to apply for relief was much reduced'.[23] 'Once an individual family or household have become acquainted with the relief machinery ... the habit of looking to poor relief as a means of subsistence becomes easy and inevitable'.[24] High unemployment levels, it was argued, had brought a large proportion of the population into contact with welfare administration; Whitehall officials gloomily surmised that applicants had found that the poor law machinery was 'not so harsh or repellent as had been anticipated'.[25]

A symptom of this kind of anxiety was the Anomalies Act of 1931. This was indeed a gendered anomaly in its 'catch 22' provision for married women: those who had left work were regarded as having retired and, supposing they were looking for work, could again be disqualified since they had no reasonable expectation of finding it.[26] In Lancashire, where women's employment had been widespread in the textile industry, half-timers were disqualified from benefit and, for those wholly unemployed, public assistance was made conditional on training programmes as a means of discouraging applications. Training was for domestic service so that women who had been the aristocrats of the female labour force were expected to do what they perceived as menial work. In Stockport, for example, there was said to be 'a definite aversion to domestic work generally and resident domestic work in particular'.[27] Even in areas where female wages had not been so high there was still a dislike of domestic work. In Sheffield, for instance, half of the women refusing employment were under 30 and one reason for their alleged voluntary unemployment was that the wage of a domestic worker did not exceed the welfare payment under the Unemployment Assessment Board, so that there was too small an inducement to work. As a result of this situation, the Board's allowance was reduced in order to increase the inducement to go into service.[28]

Service of a different kind was performed by women who acted as Poor Law Guardians, and thus managed not private households but public welfare. Within a gendered conception of citizenship the obligations of Victorian women to serve the community found a new expression after 1871 in their work as guardians. From 1881 to 1894 the Women's Guardians Society gave these isolated public women a formal, organised network of support. However, the abolition of a property qualification in 1894 resulted in a large increase in numbers of female guardians, because working-class women were now able to come forward. By 1900 there were over 1,000 female guardians, and twenty years later there were over 2,000 of them in the local state.[29] What role did female guardians play once elected? Matilda Blake, writing in 1892, spoke of the need for women to be Poor Law Guardians so that they would be able to engage in what she termed 'national housekeeping'. In her view there was 'an abundance of work which is strictly womanly', because it was both important to do justice to the female ratepayer, and to the majority of paupers who were women and children. She argued that the nature of the guardians' work was gendered, and spoke slightingly of the 'money wasted by incompetent men' who spent time discussing affairs of which they were ignorant. In Blake's view, a division of labour was preferable, so that women guardians would supervise the matron of the workhouse, take responsibility for the education and boarding out of pauper children, provide oversight of the workhouse kitchen and its production of food, as well as give attention to the conduct of confinements and the maintenance of workhouse clothing.[30] Not that all women guardians necessarily saw eye-to-eye with each other and some early propertied women were more moralistic about relief than their working-class counterparts.[31] Despite differences of approach, their achievement was far from negligible, so that Hollis has concluded that from 1875 to 1914 'much of the change in poor law policy towards the young and old, the sick, the handicapped and the fallen, was woman-led'.[32] (See also the discussion of Louisa Twining in Chapter 5.)

When women were first elected, guardians' boards were a species of masculine club and, while the public gradually accepted that a female presence on the board might be useful, no more than a token presence was called for. The *Colne and Nelson Times* (an old Liberal paper) commented in 1901, when two women stood for election locally, that: 'The contest is practically one of sex representation. ... The presence of too many women on a public body could actually embarrass the men in their very essential duties'.[33] Selena Cooper's experience during the following year in Blackburn suggests that working-class women had a particularly hard fight to get elected. She reflected, 'There is a feeling abroad that women should not enter. Their mission, people say, is to scrub floors. I have had many insults during this election'.[34]

Prejudice against women guardians did not abate, although the ways in which this was shown were later less overt. While not denying their agency in developing and modifying provisions under the poor law, this work was done under difficult conditions since the politics of gender were heavily contested. On the Manchester Public Assistance Committee one woman's experience was that 'although I rose time after time I failed to "catch the Speaker's eye" '.[35] Earlier, in Leeds, female guardians were first elected as early as 1882, and half a century later there were six women on the board including the first vice-chair, so that their position might have been expected to have become secure. However, a Leeds woman guardian was esteemed if she performed a traditional womanly role, as did Mrs Moorhouse who served for sixteen years and retired in 1919 with the accolade that

'No-one took a greater interest in the children than she did.'[36] Revealingly, in 1914 women guardians had protested about being left out of poor law delegations to London, and their male colleagues had admitted that they preferred an all-male deputation. The men said that the women took business too seriously and did not combine business with pleasure so that the men preferred to select a male foursome who would make up a card party![37] If female guardians were more assertive, they found themselves out-voted – as occurred in 1915 when they tried to get a woman appointed as assistant doctor at the poor law infirmary. They were told by the medical superintendent that, since an earlier female doctor had not been an ideal appointment, no more medical women would be chosen, and women guardians were then out-voted on this issue by their male colleagues.[38]

The poor law has not been viewed as a progressive form of welfare yet women guardians – using their authority as women and mothers – managed to influence the delivery of welfare services at the local level by helping to domesticate the workhouse, mother pauper children, and humanise the arrangements for the sick and the old. It was at local or municipal levels that women, especially Labour women, played a significant part in welfare developments during the early twentieth century.[39] And during the 1920s Labour women used the authority of their maternal and domestic experience to make a significant contribution to the local welfare of young and old, the poor and the ill through a separate-but-equal stance in the party. But during the 1930s their more integrationist stance within the Labour Party meant that in national policy debates women's special needs ceased to receive the same prominence.[40] Pat Thane has commented that Labour women before 1939 were under 'no illusions that they would benefit from significant male support' within a party that continued to be male-dominated, but still thought that gender and class were so indissolubly linked that it was preferable to work within a mainstream party rather than an all-female one. In doing so they managed to influence the welfare agenda positively at the local, if not the central level.[41] There were powerful constraints upon their sphere of action even here that inhibited them from moving beyond what were conceived as womanly concerns and, even more, from using local strength as a springboard to more general participation in national politics.

HEALTH

Given this restrictionist poor law context of much female local activism, many women's groups had campaigned for a state medical service unconnected with the poor law. There was widespread criticism of the arrangements for the new Ministry of Health in 1919 because the ministry was given responsibility for the poor law as well as for health.[42] During World War I women's organisations had been pushing with the tide in creating maternalist provision: many initiatives in infant and maternal welfare were made by the body that preceded this new Ministry, the Local Government Board, because of its concern to replace war casualties by infant lives. Indeed, these early municipal clinics have been aptly described as 'a form of war-work'. In 1914 there had been 300 municipal maternity and child welfare clinics, together with 600 health visitors for working-class mothers, but by 1918 the numbers were 700 and 2,577 respectively.[43] However, a chasm developed between the demands of women for a wide-ranging health agenda and the narrowly prescriptive health measures that meant officialdom too often hectored women for their failings as mothers. Against this, women's organisations campaigned for official recognition that female morbidity, especially that associated with childbearing, was associated with socio-economic deprivation.[44] Health, as Helen Jones has commented, was thus 'a deeply political issue' for them.[45]

The formal structures of government-subsidised infant welfare centres and schools for mothers of the early twentieth century were the lineal descendants of informal, and voluntarist maternalist provision that had taken the form of Victorian mothers' meetings.[46] During the Victorian period relatively few women had been members of friendly society schemes that catered for the health of the working class.[47] The National Health Insurance (NHI) scheme of 1911 was designed for low-income workers, and thus covered single working women and the minority of married women who were in waged work, as had the friendly societies before them. But the wives of working men were excluded from the NHI except for the payment of a maternity benefit. In 1926 the Royal Commission on Health Insurance dismissed the idea of including wives and other dependants because the cost would be 'prohibitive'.[48] The gender biases of insurance schemes meant that women were penalised by being treated alongside the men in unemployment schemes (because women had fewer claims), but in health insurance (where they had more claims), they were separated, and in 1932 their benefit rates were cut. Female MPs took exception to the official perception that married women's sickness claims under NHI were 'excessive' and that malingering had taken place. How could the state really wish to improve maternal welfare, they argued, when parliament gave a higher priority to actuarial soundness than to women's health?[49]

For the relatively few women in the NHI scheme – as for the men – the standard of care was that of an inferior class service designed for the poor. It was calculated that panel doctors could only devote three-and-a-quarter minutes to each insurance patient in the surgery, and four minutes when on visits to a patient's home.[50] (Interestingly, this is not too different from the five to six minutes provided for the patient's consultation in National Health Service (NHS) surgeries.[51]) In the first year of the new insurance system, panel practitioners on average saw two-thirds of their panel rather than the one-third that they had been expecting.[52] Official predictions had been that each insured working-class person would see their NHI panel doctor between one and two times a year, an underestimate influenced by previously low rates of contact.[53] By World War II this had risen to five contacts per year on average.[54] Since working-class female dependants were left outside the 1911 Act many of their medical conditions remained untreated because ability to pay determined whether a doctor was consulted. (See Chapter 2 where women in Meiji Japan also experienced inferior standards of health care.) In Britain married women were notorious for not incurring the expense of doctors' bills so that their health was penalised by their virtual exclusion from the NHI scheme. At the inception of the NHS in 1948 the backlog of untreated female cases – especially gynaeco-logical – was revealed.[55] Women's decisions on their consumption of health care may also have been influenced by the doctor's gender.

Whereas women guardians essentially transferred their exper-tise from the private to the public sphere and then quietly extended their role, medical women's work provided a more overt challenge to a patriarchal public sphere.[56] Female doctors posed issues of credentialism in an intra-professional struggle for power in the medical market.[57] One of the main arguments used by feminists who wanted to see medical employment opened up to women in the late nineteenth century was the central role of women patients who, it was estimated were half of those seen in general practice. The *economic* implications for male colleagues of women entrants to what was an overstocked medical market were serious and Frances Power Cobbe referred to the 'trades-unionism' of doctors in their attempts 'to keep ladies out of the lucrative profession of physician and crowd them into the ill paid one of nurses'.[58] Controlling access to education and accreditation were prime instruments for achieving occupational closure since these provided the basis for professional accreditation. The attempts by women to acquire formal medical training in the 1860s and 1870s have been well documented,[59] but less well known was continued opposition to medical women having careers. One indication of this was the tardy recognition of women as doctors in professional groups: it took until 1892 for the British Medical Association to modify its rules so that it did not exclude women,[60] and until 1908 for the Royal Colleges of Physicians and Surgeons to admit females.[61] In these circumstances it was not surprising to find Louisa Martindale MD suggesting in 1922 that the 'chief disability' of the woman GP was 'professional isolation'.[62] There was a noticeable lack of women on hospital boards, boards of examiners, and on the General Medical Council. Handbooks advising entrants to a medical career were full of professional doublespeak in discussing it as a possible career for women. In these circumstances women students at the London School of Medicine for Women were advised – not entirely ironically – that 'the first thing that women must learn is to behave like gentlemen'.[63]

Women GPs specialised in the treatment of female and child patients but few medical women were given access to general practice. Some medical women preferred other options such as work in the community. Elizabeth Garrett Anderson, when reviewing the employment of 144 women on the *Medical Register* of 1892, recognised this when she hoped that women 'had given good service to the community'.[64] Certainly, their choice of career was more limited than that of their male counterparts, and I estimate that at least one in three public appointments taken up by medical women had a paediatric or female specialism. They thus moved swiftly into expanding openings in public medical services that were so characteristic of the late nineteenth and early twentieth centuries. One of these offices was that of school medical officer. In 1908, one year after the post was created, one in eight of the total were held by women.[65] This work by medically qualified women was paralleled by related female participation in public health, although by the early twentieth century an earlier role of female sanitary inspector was being superseded by that of less well-paid health visitor.[66]

Attempts by women to gain high-status employment in medicine were often frustrated. One notorious example was that of Miss Murdoch Clark. When she was appointed in 1902 as Junior House Surgeon to the Macclesfield Infirmary six honorary surgeons resigned. After six months Clark was forced to give up her post because it proved impossible for the infirmary's surgical work to be carried on.[67] Women also endured more routine discrimination: in public health women had lower pay and worse conditions of service, while those wishing to enter general practice did so by taking assistantships at a low salary, or for room and board only.[68] Alternatively, they went to under-doctored areas such as the poorer areas of large cities, or to rural areas such as the Scottish highlands and islands. Only a minority of medical women became panel practitioners under the state's NHI scheme, and so they received a smaller percentage of their income from it than their male colleagues.[69] This was predictable since women doctors treated the women and child patients who had been almost entirely excluded from the scheme. Women GPs thus had only a small share in the substantial financial bonus that such public practice conferred on the typical male GP before 1948.

In the economically depressed inter-war period prejudices and discriminatory practices against medical women intensified. Leaders of the profession advocated non-mainstream specialisms to women such as pathology, bacteriology, electrotherapeutics, child health or nutrition.[70] The marriage bar also affected them. The best-known case was that of Dr Gladys Miall Smith, assistant medical officer for maternal and child welfare in St Pancras, who was dismissed by the borough council on her marriage in 1921. She fought back and argued that this was tantamount to confiscating her capital, but was unsuccessful in her attempts at reinstatement.[71] That marriage was a kindness to medical women was patronisingly asserted by the president of the Royal College of Physicians in 1923 since, in his view, they were better as students than doctors. As doctors, he alleged, they were prone to nervous breakdown; their conscientiousness fitted them to be subordinates rather than principals.[72] Medical women as a group were at best only tolerated rather than welcomed in their profession. Symptomatic of this was the fact that the men's medical schools that had opened their doors to women students during World War I (when there was a shortage of medical personnel) had all closed them again by 1929.

Although by World War II one in nine doctors were female, medically qualified women only gradually managed to establish themselves professionally.[73] Advancement in the profession was hard to achieve for both men and women, but particularly so for women, because strategies of professional closure meant that it was extremely difficult even to get on the first rung of the promotional ladder. In the more numerous general hospitals house posts were monopolised by men, leaving women to take up appointments in the very much smaller numbers of specialist hospitals for women and children. Women found it difficult to even observe, let alone gain practice in, specialisms like surgery. Higher hospital posts were held by members of the royal colleges and entrance to these came belatedly. For example, the first woman fellow appointed to the Royal College of Physicians was in 1934. Only exceptional women like Garrett Anderson, Aldrich Blake or Scharlieb gained the higher rungs of the profession. Interestingly, however, these successful women downplayed the issue of gender competition, and emphasised instead the importance of service and high standards for their own sake. Aldrich Blake commented to her students, 'If women are going to compete with men they must be equally efficient. . . . We talk too much about competing with men. . . . Why think about competition? If you are good at your work you are certain to succeed, and if you are not, you are certain to fail.'[74]

As we have seen earlier, female networks of both a formal and informal character helped women to sustain the pressures of the 'dual burden' and of operating in a still masculine-dominated public sphere. In professional life networks might also act as support groups for building up solidarity and an *esprit de corps*. All-female institutions such as the New Hospital for Women, founded in 1872, were important in offering posts for pioneering women in specialisms that were difficult to enter in male-dominated institutions. Female-only general practices were also useful and these often passed through generations of female principals. Professional journals such as the *Medical Women's*

Journal and the *Medical Women's Federation Newsletter* gave an opportunity for women to discuss clinical matters of interest, since sometimes they found it difficult to receive serious attention in mainstream journals. Early professional associations like the Associations of Registered Medical Women in large cities such as Glasgow, London or Manchester, or the Medical Women's Federation with its local associations, gave an opportunity for airing grievances and sharing problems.

There was a gendered division of labour in health care: men almost entirely monopolised élite hospital appointments or, as GPs, benefited financially from panel practice under the NHI, whereas medical women most frequently occupied posts in clinics that were without prospect of promotion. The perceived role of medical women as worthy but lowly workhorses was encapsulated by *The Times*:

> A great part of the burden of welfare work among the poorest is borne by medical women, who are acting as missionaries of health, and, by their unselfish toil, laying the foundations of a happier future. Their work cannot be performed by men.[75]

WELFARE STATES

Women in early- and mid-twentieth-century Britain had been regarded primarily as mothers and/or wives rather than as full citizens so that the state's interventions in health and welfare were made on the basis of a number of gendered assumptions about household roles, caring and waged work. Even in wartime, when official rhetoric apparently acknowledged – as did Winston Churchill – that women 'had definitely altered their social and sex balance which years of convention had established', any related changes in the labour market were made for 'the duration' only.[76] Earlier, despite a feminist campaign on equal pay during the 1930s which had some success in shifting attitudes, there had been no immediate practical outcome.[77] (Indeed it was not until 1954 that the decision to implement equal pay for civil servants was made.[78]) However, in 1943 equal compensation for personal injuries suffered by civilian women was achieved, and this has been saluted by H. L. Smith as 'one of the greatest victories of the feminist movement during World War II'.[79]

Two key elements in the classic welfare state of the 1940s may serve to indicate its relationship to the continuing politics of gender: first, the Beveridge Report of 1942 (and the subsequent White Paper which embodied many of its recommendations) and, second, the NHS of 1948. Beveridge's view that 'housewives as mothers have vital work to do in ensuring the adequate continuance of the British race', was heir to traditional gendered assumptions on women's role.[80] Wartime mortality in both World War I and II led to a recognition that the female maternal role was sufficiently important for an expansion of maternal health care. Under the recommendations of the Beveridge Report, for instance, an independent maternity benefit was introduced although, in general, married women were made dependent on their husband's insurance contributions. Thus the classic welfare state tended to confirm women's domestic status rather than their public equality; to look backward to their indirect participation in society as members of the family rather than recognising them as individual citizens in their own right.[81] Women were themselves divided by political allegiance, by class and by marital status and this heterogeneity meant that there was a differentiated reaction to Beveridge's welfare proposals. Many women welcomed the recognition that was given to women as mothers, as did the housewife Nella Last, who commented:

> Never, since I first listened to a speaker on the air have I felt as interested as I was by Sir William Beveridge, I'll feel a bit more hopeful about the 'brave new world' now. . . . His scheme will appeal even more to women than to men, for it is they who bear the real burden of unemployment, sickness, childbearing and rearing – and the ones who, up to now, have come off worst.[82]

Not all women were quite so uncritical. While broadly welcoming the Report as embodying some of the demands of inter-war campaigns by welfare feminists, additional suggestions were made for a lengthened welfare agenda.

The few women MPs were able to make only minor contributions to the crowded parliamentary debates on Beveridge's proposals. While appreciating the general policy thrust of the Beveridge Report, they focused critical comment on the need for payment of the child allowance to the mother (and not to the father), on the inadequacy both of maternity grants and of widows' pensions, and on the need further to consider the problems of unmarried mothers.[83] Organised women's groups showed diverse reactions. The interests of single women continued to be articulated by the National Spinsters' Pensions Association, an anti-maternalist association that had been campaigning for preferential treatment in pensions for women, as Pat Thane's chapter indicates. It argued that single women should receive pensions at 55 rather than at 60 years of age, which had already been achieved by a notable advance in 1940. Its determined secretary, Florence White, demanded to know: 'Why should they be penalised for not being married?' (In their internal Whitehall correspondence male civil servants termed White 'importunate' and 'not amenable to reason'. Despite a vigorous campaign in which branches of the Spinsters' Association sent in resolutions, individuals wrote in, and the support of twenty-three MPs was obtained, the ministry dismissively labelled it as 'the spinster pension agitation'.[84]) From an egalitarian feminist viewpoint the Women's Freedom League broadly welcomed the Beveridge Report's extension of the health service to women, and its aid to widows. But they also continued an inter-war ideological campaign in criticising it for a failure to recognise their aspiration for equal citizenship, and so 'to treat women as full and independent fellow citizens with men'.[85] Among their welfare demands was the direct insurance of married women with cash benefits if disabled, and also an independent right to a pension. In 1944 representatives from ten women's organisations combined to send a single deputation to Whitehall to discuss the Beveridge Report, which they criticised for its 'inequalities ... largely stemming from the inferior position assumed for the married woman'.[86]

Although there was little thought given to the specific needs of women in its formation, the NHS received lavish praise by contemporaries. The Minister of Health, Aneurin Bevan, remarked that 'What we are doing is being watched by the whole world. This is the biggest single experiment in the social service that the world has ever seen. We can pioneer for the world to follow.'[87] Yet the reality was somewhat different because costs outstripped expectations and so the actual standards of primary (as district from hospital) care showed little improvement from the inter-war panel system. Rather than implementing an entirely new kind of health service, the major difference was in increasing throughput so that the whole population was brought into the scheme. This was a health service with standards designed for the poor although, in a major advance, patients now included all the women as well as all the men who wished to register. Almost alone in health-care provision, however, municipal maternity and child welfare clinics remained under the local authorities so that an absence of coordination between the different sectors of the NHS continued to impede continuity in maternity care. Neither did women get free birth-control advice (for which they had campaigned for so long), until 1967.[88] (See also Chapter 6.)

The classic welfare state emerged in mid-twentieth-century Britain in an intellectual and philosophical limbo, with unanswered questions on the relationship of welfare to state power, or of the citizen's rights and obligations in the welfare state. In this context it is perhaps not surprising to note the extent to which people looked backwards towards the old world that they wished to change, rather than conceptualising the kind of new welfare system they wished to create. For example, Mrs Bessie Braddock, a Labour MP, stated that 'I think of what we are repealing, more than of what we are proposing'.[89] There was an understandable desire to abolish the poor law and eliminate its stigma, and thus to end a welfare system in which the poor received inferior treatment. The principal focus of the Labour government that enacted the welfare measures between 1945 and 1951 was on class not gender. The dominant welfare-feminism of the inter-war years had a more successful outcome in the later measures of the classic welfare state than did the less powerful equal-rights feminism. Thus it was a successful outcome for the traditional role of woman-as-mother who had responsibilities, rather than for the aspiring role of woman-for-herself who had rights.[90] Free health care in the NHS, family allowances paid to mothers, and differentiated pensions were real but understated female gains. But in other respects the welfare state of the 1940s perpetuated a politics of gender in which women failed to achieve full and equal citizenship, and in which a brave new world was only partially realised.[91]

How does this qualified outcome relate to earlier successes in maternalist policies? Enfranchisement in 1918 and 1928 did not give women sufficient power to remodel the political system and hence to implement some kind of maternalist welfare agenda. Koven and Michell have pointed out that, 'Maternalism always operated on two levels: it extolled the private virtues of domesticity while simultaneously legitimating women's public relationships.'[92] Crucially, maternalism was a precariously balanced concept which depended on external political and economic circumstances for its equilibrium point between the private and the public. And in a wider political interpretation Elshtain has concluded that women's failure to translate the vote into reforming power was predictable: suffragists wrongly thought that they could take the 'identifying terms of the private sphere ... and ramify these terms into the public sphere'. They did not recognise the realities of the power structure and its embodiment of an Aristotelian public/private split in which women were, by definition, only private persons.[93] Applying this insight to the early maternalist state in Britain reveals that its focus was on woman's function as a mother and that this did not translate automatically into a status as an individual, and thus into a citizen's role. Indeed, it was precisely because they were able to ground their policies in sexual difference, and in a perpetuation of traditionalist roles for women, that earlier proponents of maternalist policies had been able to appeal so successfully to male policy-makers. Their successes had come at the local and municipal level where a 'domesticated politics' facilitated a gendered citizenship of contribution.

British women remained rooted in family, community and locality, rather than being able as a group to effect a full transition to the public, institutionalised realm of the nation state's political life.[94] Welfare benefits in Britain remained tied to full labour market participation. Continued discrimination against women in employment, together with the impediments to continuity in the labour market that motherhood imposed, meant that many women were profoundly disadvantaged by this linkage.[95] Indeed, their moral claim to welfare benefits as mothers might effectively substitute for their political claim to welfare rights as workers. The role of women as Poor Law Guardians or health-care professionals during the early twentieth century provided illustrative case studies of this marginalisation in terms of both employment and politics.[96] It was in this context that women's demands continued to be heeded selectively. The legislation of the late 1940s was enacted by a Labour Party that was itself constructed on the basis of labour solidarity and driven by the past inequities of a capitalist society. Thus, in attempting to effect social justice in welfare when it achieved office in 1945, Labour was more sensitive to class than to gender discriminations; the latter were sufficiently pervasive in a patriarchal society to appear natural. Indeed, Pamela Graves in her study of Labour women has concluded that the welfare state enacted by a Labour ministry 'reveals hardly a trace of Labour women's input'.[97]

In stating that 'women have become ends in themselves and not merely means to the ends of men' in the development of the classic welfare state,[98] the contemporary feminist, Vera Brittain, was celebrating tangible welfare improvements. But she failed to acknowledge that these successes were partial. (See also the chapter by Jane Lewis on this point.) In mistaking the part for the whole, Brittain has been joined by some later historians in their conceptualisation of an earlier maternalist system of welfare. This historical interpretation of maternalist welfare systems has been helpful, nevertheless, in saluting the achievement of women through extending the period of welfare under consideration, shifting the emphases of welfare history from the central to the local state, and recognising that motherhood linked to a political agenda could be empowering for some women. It is important to recognise, however, that maternalism was a local welfare system rather than a welfare state, and that women did not have full citizenship within a body politic that remained paternalistic, with the result that women in mid-century Britain continued to operate within circumscribed and gender-specific roles.[99]

NOTES

1 I am extremely grateful to H. L. Smith and J. Stewart for their careful reading and perceptive comments on this chapter.
2 G. Bock and P. Thane (eds), *Maternity and Gender Policies. Women and the Rise of the European Welfare States, 1880s–1950s*, London, Routledge, 1991, pp 4–6; T. Skocpol, *Protecting Soldiers and Mothers. The Political Origins of Social Policy in the United States*, Cambridge, Mass., Harvard University Press, 1992, p. 3; S. Michel and S. Koven, 'Womanly Duties: Maternalist Policies and the Origins of Welfare States in France, Germany, Great Britain and the United States, 1880–1920', *American Historical Review*, 1990, vol. 95, p. 1077; S. Koven and S. Michel (eds), *Mothers of a New World. Maternalist Politics and the Origins of Welfare States*, London, Routledge, 1993; M. Ladd-Taylor, *Mother-Work, Women, Child Welfare and the State, 1890–1930*, Urbana and Chicago, University of Illinois Press, 1994, pp. 2–3, where maternalism is more narrowly defined than in Skocpol or Koven and Michel; Special Issue on 'Motherhood, Race and the State in the Twentieth Century' of *Gender and History*, 1992, vol. 4, no. 3; J. Lewis, 'Gender, the Family and Women's Agency in the Building of "Welfare States": the British Case', *Social History*, 1994, vol. 19.

3 S. Michel and S. Koven, 'Womanly Duties', p. 1082.
4 T. Skocpol, *Soldiers and Mothers*, pp. 51–2, 424, 465–6.
5 A. Buttafuoco, 'Motherhood as Political Strategy: The Role of the Italian
   Women's Movement in the Creation of the *Cassa Nazione di Maternita*',
   in Bock and Thane, *Maternity and Gender Policies*, pp. 178–9.
6 J. Lewis, 'Gender, the Family and Women's Agency in the Building
   of "Welfare States": the British Case', *Social History*, 1994, vol. 19,
   pp. 39–41.
7 E. Rathbone, *Milestones: Annual Presidential Addresses to the
   NUSEC*, Liverpool, 1929. Speech of 11 March 1925.
8 J. Lewis and D. Piachoud, 'Women and Poverty in the Twentieth
   Century', in C. Glendinning and J. Millar (eds), *Women and Poverty
   in Britain*, London, Harvester, 1987, pp. 28–9.
9 P. Thane, 'Women and the Poor Law in Victorian and Edwardian
   England', *History Workshop*, 1978, vol. 6, pp. 31, 49.
10 Lynn Hollen Lees, 'Survival of the Unfit in London', in P. Mandler
   (ed.), *The Uses of Charity. The Poor on Relief in the Nineteenth-
   Century Metropolis*, Philadelphia, University of Pennsylvania Press,
   1990, p. 84. See also her essay, 'Women and the Welfare Process in
   Mid-Nineteenth Century England', in A. Digby, J. Innes, R. M. Smith
   (eds), *Poverty and Relief: England from the Sixteenth to the Twentieth
   Centuries*, forthcoming, Cambridge, 1996.
11 Centre for North-West Regional Studies, University of Lancashire,
   Testimony of Mr T.B.P. (born 1886). See also, E. Ross, 'Labour and
   Love: Rediscovering London's Working Class Mothers, 1870–1918',
   in J. Lewis (ed.), *Labour and Love. Women's Experience of Home
   and Family, 1850–1940*, Oxford, Blackwell, 1986, pp. 84–8.
12 M. Bondfield, *A Life's Work*, London, Hutchinson, 1949, p. 132;
   J. Lee, *Tomorrow is a New Day*, London, Cressent Press, 1939, p. 237.
13 Centre for North-West Regional Studies, University of Lancashire,
   Testimony of Mrs M. I. P. (born 1913.)
14 E. Roberts, *A Woman's Place. An Oral History of Working-Class
   Women, 1890–1940*, Oxford, Blackwell, 1984, ch. 5.
15 H. Mitchell, *The Hard Way Up*, London, Virago, 1977, pp. 125, 204.
16 Quoted in P. Ryan, 'Poplarism, 1894–1930', in P. Thane (ed.), *The
   Origins of British Social Policy*, London, Croom Helm, 1978, p. 76.
17 Durham Record Office, U/CS/303, correspondence of Chester Le
   Street Union.
18 B. Harris, 'Unemployment, Insurance and Health in Interwar Britain',
   in B. Eichengreen (ed.), *Interwar Unemployment in International Perspective*, Dordrecht and London, Kluwer Academic, 1988, pp. 149,
   166.
19 M. A. Crowther, 'Family Responsibility and State Responsibility in
   Britain before the Welfare State', *Historical Journal*, 1982, vol. 25,
   p. 145.
20 W. H. Beveridge, *The Past and Present of Unemployment Insurance*,
   Oxford, Clarendon Press, 1930, p. 24.
21 PRO, MH 57/97E Sir Arthur Robinson (Assistant Secretary) to the
   minister.

22 PRO, T 172/1584, MH 57/97E, Inspectors reports by Francis and Hughes-Gibb.
23 PRO, MH 57/97, Poor law general inspectors reports, 1928–9.
24 PRO, MH 57/207, Investigation into outrelief, Memorandum Feb. 1933.
25 PRO, MH 57/8, Public assistance conference, 1935.
26 J. Lewis, 'Dealing with Dependency: State Practices and Social Realities, 1870–1948', in J. Lewis (ed.), *Women's Welfare/Women's Rights*, London, Croom Helm, 1983, p. 27.
27 PRO, AST 12/38, Manchester Unemployment Assistance Board District 1, 1938 Enquiry.
28 PRO, AST12/34, Regional Unemployment Assistance Board Officers Reports, 1937.
29 P. Hollis, *Ladies Elect. Women in English Local Government, 1865–1914*, Oxford, Clarendon Press, 1987, p. 486.
30 M. M. Blake, 'Women as Poor Law Guardians', *Westminster Review*, 1893, vol. 139, pp. 12–21.
31 Hollis, *Ladies Elect*, p. 238.
32 Hollis, *Ladies Elect*, p. 282.
33 *Colne and Nelson Times*, 22 March 1901.
34 J. Liddington, *The Life and Times of a Respectable Rebel. Selena Cooper 1864–1946*, London, Virago, 1984, p. 131.
35 Mitchell, *Hard Way*, p. 214.
36 *Leeds Mercury*, 11 January 1919.
37 *Leeds Mercury*, 4 July 1914.
38 *Leeds Mercury*, 25 March 1915.
39 C. Collett, *For Labour and for Women. The Women's League, 1906–18*, Manchester, Manchester University Press, 1989, pp. 186–7.
40 P. M. Graves, *Labour Women. Women in British Working Class Politics, 1918–1939*, Cambridge, Cambridge University Press, 1994, pp. 179, 217–19.
41 P. Thane, 'Women in the British Labour Party and the Construction of State Welfare, 1906–1939', in Koven and Michel (eds), *Mothers*, 1993, pp. 348, 353, 372.
42 *The People's Yearbook and Annual of the English and Scottish Wholesale Societies*, Manchester, Co-operative Wholesale Society Publications, 1924, p. 34.
43 J. M. Winter, *The Great War and the British People*, London, Macmillan, 1985, pp. 190–6; D. Dwork, *War is Good for Babies and Other Young Children. A History of the Infant and Child Welfare Movement in England, 1898–1918*, London, Tavistock, 1987, p. 211; Hollis, *Ladies*, p. 439; J. Liddington, *The Life and Times of a Respectable Rebel. Selina Cooper, 1864–1946*, London, Virago, 1984, pp. 214–15.
44 J. Lewis, 'Mothers and Maternity Policies in the Twentieth Century', in J. Garcia, R. Kilpatrick and M. Richards (eds), *The Politics of Maternity Care. Services for Childbearing Women in Twentieth-Century Britain*, Oxford, Clarendon Press, 1990, pp. 23–4.
45 H. Jones, *Health and Society in Twentieth Century Britain*, London, Croom Helm, 1994, p. 12.

46 F. Prochaska, 'A Mother's Country: Mother's Meetings and Family Welfare in Britain, 1850–1950', *History*, 1989, vol. 74, pp. 393–4.
47 P. H. J. H. Gosden, *The Friendly Societies of England, 1815–1875*, Manchester, Manchester University Press, 1961, pp. 61–2; F. M. L. Thompson (ed.), *The Cambridge Social History of Britain*, III, Cambridge, Cambridge University Press, pp. 431–2.
48 *Royal Commission on Health Insurance*, PP 1926, XIV, pp. 162, 314.
49 J. Lewis, *The Politics of Motherhood*, London, Croom Helm, 1980, p. 50.
50 *Medical World*, 9 April 1914.
51 E. Balint and J. S. Norell, *Six Minutes for the Patient. Interactions in General Practice Consultations*, Tavistock Mind and Medicine Monograph 23, 1973.
52 *Medical World*, 9 April 1914.
53 PRO, MH 77/182, Evidence to Spens Committee by Bradford Hill and BMA.
54 A. Digby and N. Bosanquet, 'Doctors and Patients in an Era of National Health Service and Private Practice, 1911–1938', *Economic History Review*, second series, 1988, vol. XLI, p. 87.
55 Roberts, *A Woman's Place*, p. 107.
56 See A. Digby, *Making a Medical Living. Doctors and Patients in the English Market for Medicine, 1720–1911*, Cambridge, Cambridge University Press, 1994, ch. 9 for a fuller discussion of this issue.
57 A. Witz, 'Patriarchy and the Professions: the Gendered Politics of Occupational Closure', *Sociology*, 1990, vol. 24, pp. 675–90. See also E. Fox, 'An Honourable Calling or a Despised Occupation: Licensed Midwifery and its Relationship to District Nursing in England and Wales before 1948', *Social History of Medicine*, 1993, vol. 6, pp. 237–60 for a discussion of wider strategies of inter-occupational closure at work.
58 Cobbe, 'Medicine and Morality', p. 323.
59 For example, J. Manton, *Elizabeth Garrett Anderson*, London, Methuen, 1965; E. Moberley Bell, *Storming the Citadel*, 1953; P. Chambers, *A Doctor Alone: A Biography of Elizabeth Blackwell*, London, Bodley Head, 1956.
60 It had admitted inadvertently E. Garrett Anderson and then altered the regulations in 1878 so as to specifically prohibit women.
61 *Medical Women's Journal*, 1908, vol. 18, p. 258.
62 L. Martindale, *The Woman Doctor and her Future*, London, Mills & Boon, 1922, p. 85.
63 Garrett Anderson's dictum as Dean of the School, quoted in Manton, *Garrett Anderson*, p. 311.
64 *Westminster Review*, March 1893.
65 *Annual Report of the Chief Medical Officer of the Board of Education for 1910*, Cd 5426, PP 1910, XXIII, pp. 192–3.
66 C. Davies, 'The Health Visitor as Mother's Friend: A Woman's Place in Public Health, 1900–1914', *Social History of Medicine*, 1988, vol. 1, p. 57.
67 *Women's Medical Journal*, 1902, vol. 12, p. 8.

68 *Women's Medical Journal*, 1921, vol. 28, p. 307; *Medical Women's Federation Newsletter*, July 1928, pp. 85–6.
69 *Lancet*, 5 May 1923, p. 984.
70 *Lancet*, ii, 1926, pp. 740–2; *BMJ*, ii, 1925, p. 43; *BMJ*, ii, 1927, p. 416.
71 *The Times*, 20 October 1921; *Medical Officer*, 1921, vol. 26, p. 56.
72 *Lancet*, ii, 1923, pp. 765–8. Address by Sir H. Rolleston at the Royal Free Hospital.
73 *Royal Commission on Equal Pay, Minutes of First Day's Evidence*, 1945, Appendix, p. 187. (Based on a survey by the BMA of 1937.)
74 Lord Riddell, *Dame Louisa Aldrich-Blake*, London, Hodder & Stoughton, 1926, p. 43.
75 Leader in *The Times*, 3 October 1924.
76 H. L. Smith, 'The Womanpower Problem in Britain during the Second World War', *Historical Journal*, 1984, vol. 27, pp. 925, 945.
77 H. L. Smith, 'British Feminism and the Equal Pay Issue in the 1930s', forthcoming, *Women's History Review* (1995). I am most grateful to the author for allowing me to see this before publication.
78 H. L. Smith, 'The Politics of Conservative Reform: the Equal Pay for Equal Work Issue, 1945-1955', *Historical Journal*, 1992, vol. 35, pp. 405–15.
79 H. L. Smith, 'The Problem of "Equal Pay for Equal Work" in Great Britain during World War II', *Journal of Modern History*, 1981, vol. 53, p. 663.
80 *Report on Social Insurance and Allied Services*, PP 1942, Cmd 6404, VI, p. 53.
81 S. Pedersen, 'Gender, Welfare and Citizenship during the Great War', *American History Review*, 1990, vol. 95, p. 984; E. DuBois, 'The Radicalism of the Woman's Suffrage Movement', in A. Phillips (ed.), *Feminism and Equality*, Oxford, Blackwell, 1987, p. 131.
82 R. Board and S. Fleming (eds), *Nella Last's War*, Bristol, Falling Wall Press, 1983, p. 227.
83 *Hansard*, 16–18 February, 386, cols 1667, 1781, 1791–4, 2021 (contributions of Rathbone (Independent), Cazalet Keir (Conservative), and Adamson (Labour) to debates on 16 to 18 February 1943).
84 PRO, PIN 8/69, Undated memorandum from F. White to Sir W. Jowett, Minister Designate of Social Security.
85 E. Abbott and K. Bompas, *The Woman Citizen*, London, K. Bompas, 1943, p. 18.
86 PRO, PIN 8/48, Deputation to discuss Beveridge Report.
87 Speech, 7 October 1948, Frontispiece in C. Webster (ed.), *Aneurin Bevan on the National Health Service*, Oxford, Wellcome Unit for the History of Medicine Research Publication X, 1991.
88 Crucially, the NHS (Family Planning) Act 1967 enabled local authorities to give contraceptive advice on social as well as medical grounds, without restrictions as to age or marital status. (A. Leathard, *The Fight for Family Planning. The Development of Family Planning Services in Britain 1921–1974*, London, Macmillan, 1980.)
89 *Hansard*, 4 July 1948, 444, col. 1631.
90 See D. Riley, *Am I that Name? Feminism and the Category of 'Women'*

in History, London, Macmillan, 1988, p. 40; and M. Molloy, 'Citizenship, Property and Bodies: Discourses on Gender and the Inter-war Labour Government in New Zealand', *Gender and History*, 1993, vol. 4, p. 301 for a fuller discussion of this distinction.

91   J. Dale, 'Feminists and the Development of the Welfare State – Some Lessons from our History', *Critical Social Policy*, 1986, vol. 16, pp. 57–65.

92   Koven and Michel, 'Womanly Duties', p. 1079.

93   J. B. Elshtain, 'Aristotle, the Public-Private Split, and the Case of the Suffragists', in J. B. Elshtain (ed.), *The Family in Political Thought*, Brighton, Harvester, 1982, p. 58.

94   C. C. Gould, 'Private and Public Virtues: Women, the Family and Democracy', in C. C. Gould, *Beyond Domination: New Perspectives on Women and Philosophy*, Totowa, New Jersey, Roman & Allanheld, 1983, pp. 16–18.

95   See J. Colwill, 'Beveridge and the Welfare State', *Critical Social Policy*, 1994, vol. 41, pp. 53–78, for a critique of the gender discrimination inherent in a contributory rather than benefit entitlement scheme.

96   In 'Gender, the Family', p. 55, Jane Lewis makes the important point that in the longer term labour market participation in the welfare state itself provided for the possibility of female agency.

97   Graves, *Labour Women*, p. 220.

98   V. Brittain, *Lady into Woman. A History of Women from Victoria to Elizabeth II*, London, Andrew Dakers, 1953, p. 224.

99   Whether a universalised welfare system implied a potential enhancement of women's future agency in the longer term remains a contentious issue that lies outside the remit of this paper. See, for example, the arguments of H. Hernes, *Welfare State and Woman Power: Essays in State Feminism*, Oslo, Oslo University Press, 1987, and J. E. Kolberg, 'The Gender Dimension of the Welfare State', *International Journal of Sociology*, 1991, vol. XXI.

Chapter 4

Octavia Hill and women's networks in housing

Caroline Morrell

Octavia Hill (1838–1912) was one of the outstanding figures of Victorian social reform. Her fame has faded somewhat today, but she was a household name in her own lifetime, and her influence spread well into the twentieth century. In 1942 Sir Reginald Rowe, president of the National Federation of Housing Societies, said of her: 'I doubt if in the fields of human service there has been any other woman who has sown seeds from which so much has grown and is still growing.'[1] Written thirty years after Hill's death, this reflects the standing in which she was held by her immediate successors. Her reputation derived from her work in the field of working-class housing and her role in the establishment of the National Trust. But she also played a prominent part in other movements of the time and achieved the status of a national expert on social issues. She was a remarkable woman who achieved her reputation on the strength of her work, and as such she was one of a group of Victorian women who forged careers in the public world and showed by their example that women could successfully step out of their traditional role. This could not have been an easy path to follow, so this chapter will investigate the support mechanisms which enabled women such as Octavia Hill to perform their new roles in the public sphere. Octavia operated through an extensive network of family, friends and colleagues which overlapped in several areas, and the focus will be on this network and the role it played in sustaining her in her work. Networks are made up of personal relationships and those that existed between Octavia Hill and her sisters, friends and co-workers will be discussed while I shall look in particular detail at her relationships with two significant women friends, Sophia Jex-Blake and Harriot Yorke.

Human relationships, while easy to talk about and fascinating to speculate about, are in essence slippery, intangible, insubstantial and difficult to pin down. Consisting as they do of emotions and feelings, they lack any physical substance and only leave behind historical traces in letters and diaries. It is difficult enough to be objective about our own relationships, even more difficult to talk with any certainty about those of other people, and perhaps arrogant to assume that one can have any real insight into the relationships of people one has never met and who are, after all, dead. Only those who were involved in the relationships can really know what they meant. For the historian all this is complicated by the fact that the evidence that is left is inevitably second- or third-hand, feelings filtered through and distorted by the very act of writing about them, letters and diaries which may have been edited and censored. We know that some of Octavia's letters were destroyed on her orders and that others were suppressed by her family,[2] so at best we get a selective and selected view. It is also easy to misread and misinterpret the evidence we have, and to overlay it with our own preconceptions and preoccupations. Yet with all these reservations, I think that it is important to pay attention to, and try to understand, the personal relationships of historical figures. They are not, I think, secondary or minor, or essentially private aspects of a person's life, but can tell us a great deal about that person's public life and work. This is particularly true of nineteenth-century women, as their exclusion from the public world meant that their family and friends perhaps played a much more important part in their lives than they did for men. Women's lives tended to be constructed out of relationships with other people so that they were identified as wives, mothers, daughters at home, or maiden aunts, rather than as actors in their own right. And this remains important in women's lives today.

Such women as Octavia Hill found their identity in ways other than through marriage or children. Octavia became famous on the strength of her work, yet I would argue that for her, her personal relationships with other women were of critical importance in enabling her to carry out this role as a public person. They provided her with both domestic support at home and the emotional support necessary in forging a new career. In many ways this broke the conventions of what a woman's role should be. Octavia chose to live all her life with other women, she worked with women and, to a large extent in her housing and social work, she worked for women, and she placed immense importance on her relationships with women in all those spheres. She was a pioneer, an outstanding public figure, and one of the questions that I would like to ask in this chapter is, 'What made her so effective?' Did her relationships with other women play a role in her public success, and could she have operated so effectively without these sustaining relationships?

The role of networks in Victorian society and the way that they operated in connection with the rise of a new class of 'intellectual aristocracy' has been identified by Noel Annan.[3] In an influential essay, he traced the connections of marriage which existed between a number of radical, evangelical and academic families in Victorian England and showed how a few families, through their multifarious links, came to dominate academic and intellectual life in Britain. Jane Rendall makes connections between these families, particularly those of a Unitarian or Quaker persuasion – which retained 'something of an older, egalitarian outlook towards the relations between men and women'[4] – and the emergence of the nineteenth-century movement for women's rights. Feminist historians have become increasingly interested in the significance of women's networks and the role they played in the development of the early women's movement. Ray Strachey,[5] in her early history of the women's movement in Britain, records the activities of a vast number of women campaigners and organisations and details the complex nature of the connections which existed between them. More recent feminist historians have also focused on the friendship networks which existed between women. Martha Vicinus, in her work on single women in the nineteenth century, writes of 'a network of women's organisations and institutions [which] supported each single woman entering the newly developing professions for women.'[6] Liz Stanley,[7] in her work on feminist biography, has also focused on the networks which surrounded particular historical figures. Rather than the traditional biography of the 'great woman', with its spotlight on the individual, she advocates 'a more complex portrayal of them as a friend among friends, a colleague among colleagues'.[8] 'An approach to biography informed by feminism and sociology', she further argues, 'should recognise that these connexions, social networks, call them what you will, are a crucial means of enabling us to appreciate and understand past, and present, lives and achievements.' Philippa Levine,[9] in her work on Victorian feminists, has adopted a similar approach. Taking a sample of 196 women active in various women-centred campaigns, she has formulated a collective biography, a prosopography of feminism in the period *c.* 1850–*c.* 1900, identifying 'a strong network of activity and support, which promoted deep and sustained friendships among women'.[10] Such mapping of networks then can help us place an individual in context, and it can also go some way towards retrieving the lives of many other women. These 'unsung heroines' of the women's movement have been overshadowed by their more celebrated sisters. It is the nature and quality of the relationships which formed these networks which particularly interests me, and Octavia Hill with her extensive circle of friends, wide range of activities and, importantly, the wealth of letters she left behind, provides an example of how this networking operated in one particular woman's case.

Housing is the area in which Octavia made her reputation and it would be useful to give a brief sketch of her achievements in this field. It was John Ruskin who launched Octavia in her career in housing, and it is important to remember that Octavia enjoyed the support and friendship of men throughout her career. Octavia first met Ruskin in the early 1850s when she was working as superintendent of a class of ragged school children in the Ladies Guild, a Co-operative venture managed by her mother. Ruskin offered to train her as a copyist of illuminated manuscripts and Old Masters, and she spent over ten years as his pupil and protégée. They developed a close relationship and Octavia was deeply influenced by his ideas not only on art, but also on religion, society and nature.[11] When Ruskin's father died in 1864, leaving him a large amount of money, he offered to help Octavia begin a new experiment in housing the poor. He bought the lease of three houses in Paradise Place, a rundown court near her home in Marylebone, for her to manage. Octavia was to rehabilitate the houses and run them on humane lines while returning a small amount of interest on the investment. Both were determined to prove that working-class housing could be run decently and still return a profit, and hoped that by their example other landlords would be persuaded to take up their methods. Octavia was successful in this first venture, and the following year Ruskin bought the lease of another court in Freshwater Place. From here Octavia went on to run many other housing schemes in London and to employ women housing workers on a large scale.

What was different about Octavia's methods of housing management was that she believed in rehabilitation – of both buildings and tenants – and that she cared as much for the welfare of her tenants as for the bricks and mortar. Up to this point most working-class housing had been managed on the principle of rent collection and eviction with the extraction of maximum profit as the overriding motive. The consequent overcrowding and disease evoked the response of wide-scale slum clearance, and the new type of model dwellings intended to provide decent and afford-able housing for the labouring classes. This, far from alleviating the problem, resulted in the displacement of slum-dwellers, and many thousands more people being made homeless.[12] Octavia saw clearly that effective housing management could not be based upon building alone, but also required care for the tenants: 'You cannot deal with the people and their houses separately', she said, 'the principle on which the whole work rests, is that the inhabitants and their surroundings must be improved together'.[13] And it is here that she made her special mark – she created a system of housing management which rested upon the gradual improvement of both tenants and housing, and strove to achieve caring communities of responsible, rent-paying tenants. The regular payment of rent and the maintenance of standards of good housekeeping were rewarded by material improvements to her tenants' homes, but over and above this, a whole design for living was incorporated into Octavia's housing schemes. She provided playgrounds for the children (with paid supervisors); saving clubs and employment schemes; workshops, classes, gardens and social clubs for her tenants; and took them on trips to the countryside and arranged regular festivities and entertainments. Her attention to the details of people's lives must have made her schemes much more pleasant and human places to live than the big blocks built by the model dwelling companies. Simple touches, such as the bringing up of bunches of flowers from the countryside for her tenants, demonstrate the care she took over every aspect of their lives, and show a distinctly feminine approach to the business of housing management.

The hallmark of her system was the personal and individual nature of the relationship between the lady rent-collector and the tenants, and she adamantly believed that women were better suited to this than men. 'Ladies must do it,' she said, 'for it is detailed work; ladies must do, it for it is household work.'[14] She ran her early schemes with the help of her sisters and friends, but as the work expanded more women became involved – some in a voluntary capacity, some as paid workers. By 1874 Octavia had fifteen housing schemes under her care containing between two and three thousand tenants[15] and enough workers to begin her annual letter to fellow workers. Her work expanded over the next thirty years to include a large number of housing schemes in London, some consisting of just a few properties in a court or street, but others comparatively large, such as the estates in south London which Octavia managed on behalf of the Ecclesiastical Commissioners. Walworth Estate, for example, Octavia's largest estate, covered twenty-two acres and had between five and six hundred houses.[16] We do not know exactly how much property Octavia managed or how many workers were involved as Octavia kept no definitive list. Some idea of the scale of her work is given in a pamphlet issued by the Society of Women Housing Managers in 1946: 'At the time of her death in 1912, she directly controlled over two thousand tenancies [representing perhaps some ten thousand individuals] and a number of women managers trained in her system were at work, not only in England and Scotland, but in Sweden, Holland and the United States.'[17]

Octavia achieved an international reputation in the field of housing, but she was also active in other social movements. She was a founder member of the Charity Organisation Society (COS), an association set up in the 1860s to coordinate and rationalise the relief activities of charities with that of the poor law, and through her work with the COS helped develop the methods of individual investigation and case-work which formed the basis of future social work training. She was also closely involved in the first Women's University Settlement, set up in Southwark in 1889, and many of these early women settlers spent part of their training helping in Octavia's housing schemes. Her concern about the cramped lives of her urban tenants led her into the Open Spaces movement, aimed at preserving areas of open land for the enjoyment of the poor, and in 1895 she was one of the three founders of the National Trust. Octavia was regarded as an expert on housing and social affairs, and in 1884 was called as one of the chief witnesses to the Royal Commission on the Housing of the Working Classes. She was also one of the three women members of the Royal Commission on the Poor Law, alongside Beatrice Webb and Helen Bosanquet. The standing in

which she was held in her own lifetime is reflected by the fact
that in 1887 she was one of only three women to be invited in
their own right to Queen Victoria's Golden Jubilee Service (the
others being Josephine Butler and Florence Nightingale)[18] and
that on her death her family was offered a funeral in Westminster
Abbey.[19] They refused this honour and the service was held
instead in Southwark Cathedral.

Octavia Hill was an outstanding woman who demonstrated
that women could be successful and effective in the public world,
and as such she must have acted as both a role model and an
inspiration to Victorian women looking for a new role in the
world. As Jane Lewis[20] points out, she was involved in the three
areas of social work in which so many women started their
working lives outside the home: the COS, housing management
and settlement work. Octavia helped pioneer the movement of
women out of the private sphere of home, family and unpaid
charity work into the public world. By her example she was a
feminist, but it was not a label that she ever claimed for herself.
I had initially hoped to find some evidence of a feminist campaign
based around housing, and perhaps to claim Octavia as a pioneer
of the early women's movement. It seemed to me that housing
and the home are so central to the lives of women, and that
Victorian women of all classes were so dependent on men for
housing, that women activists of the day must have made some
connections between women's unequal housing conditions and
women's unequal position in society in general and identified it
as a cause to become involved in. But Octavia was a very complex,
and in some ways parodoxical, figure, and not one easy to pin a
label on. She supported some women's causes, but not others. She
was active, for example, in the campaign for married women's
property rights and for higher education for women, but she was
adamantly opposed to women's suffrage. In 1910 she wrote to *The
Times* to say: 'I feel I must say how profoundly sorry I shall be
if women's suffrage in any form is introduced into England.'[21]
When Lord Cromer approached her to ask her to add her name
to an anti-suffrage letter she replied: 'the very thing which makes
me feel how fatal it would be for women to be drawn into the
political arena precludes my signing the letter and joining in what
must be a political campaign.'[22] This is interesting coming from
someone who was, in fact, very active in the political world,
advising government ministers and lobbying, very effectively,

for legislative change. Her sister Miranda wrote of Octavia's activities in the lobbying processes surrounding the question of the preservation of open spaces:

> It *has* come to a point! – when two peers and a cabinet minister call and consult her in one week. She had Fawcett here yesterday, Lord Wemyss the day before to ask what he should say in the House of Lords and the Duke of Westminster on Wednesday to ask what the Prince of Wales could do in the matter.[23]

Octavia *was* a political person, and her opposition to women's suffrage at first glance seems at odds with the rest of her life. It was not that she did not believe that women had a right to a role in the public world, but she held an essentially gendered view of citizenship, in which the roles of men and women were complementary. As women were so eminently suited to the sphere of the home, family and the local community, they should not waste their special skills in the world of national politics – the sphere of men. She argued, therefore, that: 'I believe that men and women help one another because they are different, have different gifts and different spheres, one is the complement of the other.'[24] These forcefully held views did not prevent Octavia from having close friendships and working relationships with women who were just as strongly in favour of women's suffrage. Many of Octavia's friends and associates were committed suffragists, and this transcending of political differences seems to have been a feature of women's activities of the time. Pro- or anti-suffrage, radical or liberal, women worked together on issues such as access to education or employment, married women's property rights or moral reform, and links of friendship, or sisterhood, seemed in most cases more important than perfect convergence of views.

Octavia's greatest contribution to the women's movement was her creation of a new career for women, that of housing management. But while she was very effective in seizing housing as women's work, she did so on the grounds of women's special duty to the home and the family, and she talked very much more in terms of women's duties than women's rights. She lauded the values of home and family life and the roles of wife and mother:

> Is not she most sympathetic, most powerful, who nursed her own mother through her long illness, and knew how to go quietly about the darkened room; who entered so heartily into

her sister's love and marriage; who obeyed so perfectly the father's command when it was hardest? Better still, if she be a wife and mother herself, and can enter into the responsibilities of a head of household, understand her joys and cares, knows what heroic patience it needs to keep gentle when the nerves are unhinged and the children noisy.[25]

Octavia did nurse various members of her family through illnesses and she did rejoice in her sisters' marriages, but she certainly did not conform to the rest of this homily. She never married, had no children, and, far from living in a conventional family home, lived all her life in a shared household of women – her mother, sisters, companion and other workers. As for her father's hard commands, she had none to obey because he lived separately from his family. (James Hill, Octavia's father, suffered a mental breakdown following a series of business failures in the early 1840s and on medical advice moved away from his family.) All this does make one wonder what Octavia made of her position as a single woman, and whether she considered the single life second best? Possibly she sublimated all sorts of repressed feelings in her work, but she certainly seems to have led a rich emotional life without a husband or children, particularly through her relationships with other women. She also had warm friendships with men: she was fond of her brothers-in-law, Charles Lewis and Edmund Maurice, and worked closely with male colleagues in the various campaigns with which she was involved. She was also engaged briefly to Edward Bond, a lawyer, who worked with her throughout the 1870s in committees connected with her housing schemes and the Open Spaces movement. In 1877, when Octavia was 39 and Bond six years younger, they became engaged, but the engagement was broken off almost immediately, apparently on the opposition of his mother.

Octavia's network was a wide one and as I read through, first, Gillian Darley's detailed biography of Octavia, and then the published volumes of Octavia's letters, what caught my attention were the same names which cropped up time and time again, not all necessarily connected with housing. Octavia had friends and contacts in many different areas, ranging from childhood friends to members of the royal family, and in the course of her many activities she came into contact with a host of famous nineteenth-century individuals: John Ruskin, of course, Frederick Denison Maurice, Charles Kingsley, George Eliot, Lord Shaftesbury,

William Morris, Florence Nightingale, Charles Booth, Sir Leslie
Stephen, Thomas Hughes, Beatrice Webb, Emily Davies, Barbara
Leigh Smith (Bodichon) are just a few of the names that figure
in her letters. Her spheres of activity and interest encompassed
many different movements and issues – housing, the Charity
Organisation, the Women's University Settlement, Open Spaces,
smoke-abatement, Christian Socialism, Co-operativism, art, youth
work and education. Octavia would probably not have seen any
of these activities as separate from each other; they all formed
part of her overall philosophy. Friends and colleagues from one
area of her life tended to appear in several others and, as in many
people's lives, friends, colleagues and relatives all came together
to form an intricate and complex web.

Octavia was not particularly well-connected by birth. Her
father's early bankruptcy meant that most of her childhood was
spent in relative poverty – she and her sisters had to work for
their living from an early age and the family had to take in lodgers
at various periods. Her maternal grandfather, though, was the
eminent sanitary reformer Dr Southward Smith. He worked
closely with colleagues such as Lord Shaftesbury (with whom
Octavia was later to work on the Central Committee of the COS)
and Edwin Chadwick, and was also a friend of Jeremy Bentham.
Her mother, Caroline Hill, was a noted educationalist and a
follower of Co-operativism and Christian Socialism. So although
materially poor, Octavia grew up in an interesting family milieu.
The marriages of her sisters Gertrude and Emily also brought
influential people into the family circle. Gertrude married Charles
Lewes, the stepson of George Eliot, and Emily married Edmund
Maurice, the son of Frederick Denison Maurice, the leading figure
of the Christian Socialist movement. Maurice was also active in
the movement to extend education to working men and women
and in 1856 gave Octavia the post of secretary to the women's
classes at the Working Men's College which he founded. Ruskin
taught at this school along with Llewellyn Davies, Thomas
Hughes, George MacDonald, Frederick Furnivall and other
leading members of the Christian Socialist circle. Octavia acted
as governess for a short period to Thomas Hughes' children,[26] and
became a close friend of his sister, Jane Nassau Senior. Through
her work as a teacher she was also in contact with Emily Davies,
Llewellyn Davies' sister, and in 1864 helped her collect signatures
for the petition to open university examinations to girls.[27]

It seems that there was a wide network of family friends and associates which overlapped at many points. I was particularly intrigued to discover the multi-layered relationships which existed between Octavia and three other women in this network – Barbara Leigh Smith (Bodichon), Florence Nightingale and George Eliot. Octavia knew Barbara Leigh Smith from her childhood, worked with her in her campaign to secure married women's property rights, and also taught for a while in the Portman Hall School which Barbara ran with her friend Elizabeth Whitehead Malleson. Florence Nightingale was a cousin of Barbara Bodichon and her nursing pupils were, from time to time, taken on tours of Octavia's housing schemes.[28] George Eliot was a close friend of Barbara Bodichon and, as we have seen, related to Octavia through marriage. She was an admirer of Octavia's work and contributed to her housing schemes. Her portrait of Dorothea Brooke in *Middlemarch* is said to have struck Florence Nightingale as having been modelled on Octavia.[29] Similar relationships can also be mapped between Octavia and many of the other women whom she knew, and each of these women had links with other women in the network which existed independently of her. Liz Stanley[30] points out, for example, that Barbara Leigh Smith and George Eliot were also close friends of Mary Howitt, the feminist writer and anti-slavery campaigner, with whom Octavia had a close, almost daughter-like, relationship.

Networks by their nature are not static – interests change and new friends are made – and it is difficult to give a definitive picture of a network in operation, or to say that any one person was at the centre of it. Octavia Hill is the focal point of the network I have investigated, but there are many other strands that could be followed to which she would appear peripheral. I think it is true to say though that she was the centre of the network of housing workers. It was she who pioneered this method of working, and to whom other workers came to be trained, and whose methods were copied world wide. Henrietta Barnett and Emma Cons, the other two women who worked on a large scale in housing in London, both began their careers as housing workers with Octavia, and both went on to great achievements in their own right. Henrietta Barnett was responsible for the creation of Hampstead Garden Suburb and Emma Cons, among other things, began both the Old Vic and Morley College for Working Men and Women.

The network of women housing managers was wide. I have so far been able to identify thirty-six housing schemes which were connected with Octavia in some way, and sixty-seven women who worked in housing schemes associated with Octavia or her colleagues, Emma Cons and Henrietta and Samuel Barnett. This must be an underestimate as the long span of Octavia's career in housing (over fifty years), and the size of some of the schemes, means that several hundred women must have been involved. The network also stretched overseas, and women came from Holland, Sweden and America to train with Octavia. Typically, Octavia underplayed her role in this network. In her evidence to the Royal Commission on the Housing of the Working Classes in 1884 she said:

> Eight years ago I did a great deal of decentralising, instead of aggregating to myself. I have at least five distinct centres in London: people are buying land and training workers, and enlisting volunteers, whose names and places I do not know; it does not really at all depend on me.[31]

Octavia established no formal housing organisation and refused to have any block of buildings named after her. She was adamant her way of working was not to be crystallised and that she herself should not be seen as the lynch-pin of it. Towards the end of her life she said:

> When I am gone, I hope my friends will not try to carry out any special system, or to follow blindly in the track which I have trodden. New circumstances require various efforts; and it is the spirit, not the dead form, that should be perpetuated.[32]

However, after her death a number of her workers came together to form the Society of Women Housing Estate Managers in order to carry on her methods, and in 1928 Miss Jefferey, one of her later workers, formed the Octavia Hill Club from among the women she had trained.[33]

The way that this informal network operated shows women networking in a very practical way. Individuals came to Octavia to be trained – she would place them in one of her own schemes or recommend them to another housing manager, and workers moved between schemes. Sisters brought in sisters and friends other friends. Catherine Potter, for example, first worked with

Octavia and then moved over to the Barnetts to work in one of their housing schemes in the East End. Henrietta Barnett said of her: 'For eight years Miss Potter worked with us, bringing in her wake her hosts of friends, as well as two sisters, Miss Theresa ... [and] Miss Beatrice'[34] (later to become Beatrice Webb). Elizabeth Sturge, who came from Bristol to work with Octavia in 1886, did so following a meeting with an old school friend, Anna Hogg, who was at that point working with Octavia in Deptford.[35]

The benefactors of Octavia's schemes were also part of a wider network. Some of them, such as the Sterling sisters, had known Octavia from her days working as secretary to the women's classes at the Working Men's College. Some such, as the Davenport-Hill sisters, were COS colleagues. Some, such as Mrs Russell-Gurney and William Shaen (Octavia's solicitor), were old friends. And, significantly, in many cases friendships and business relationships became identical. Octavia, for example, developed a close friendship with Lady Ducie, who provided property for various of her schemes and worked with her over a long period. She invited her to her country house for recuperative breaks to recover from the stresses of work, and took a close interest in Octavia's health. Friends and benefactors joined together in 1874 to set up a fund to release Octavia from the necessity of earning a living through teaching in order that she might concentrate solely on her housing work.

As well as having networks, women could also 'network' in an instrumental way. In 1869, for example, Octavia was hoping to be nominated to the first COS committee to be set up in her parish in Marylebone. 'Mr F., the rector of our district and the main mover in the matter, is to call on me today,' she wrote to a friend, '... I shall try boldly: but I think no ladies will be admitted. Mr F. is happily a friend of Lady Ducie's.'[36] Octavia was duly nominated, and she then nominated her friend and trainee Henrietta Barnett to the committee. Henrietta's brother-in-law, Ernest Hart, came to Octavia's aid when in 1874 she was running into difficulties with the local medical officer of health over the condition of her houses in Barrett's Court. He was the editor of the *British Medical Journal*, and his intervention persuaded the medical officer to drop the case.[37]

These links show very clearly the complex and overlapping nature of the networks in which Octavia was involved. It does not seem possible to separate out the links of personal friendship and family relationships from those of work, but I think that this is very characteristic of the women's movement of the time. It can be seen as an example of a particular way of working which could be said to be peculiarly 'feminine', or perhaps 'feminist'. The central role which these women played in each other's lives, and the support and encouragement they gave each other, were critical to the development of the women's movement. And the way in which Octavia related to other women is as important as her public achievements in defining her status as a feminist. In other words when we are discussing feminism, process is as important as aims.

Octavia had something of a talent for friendship. She sustained life-long correspondences and clearly placed a great deal of value on her friends. Her closest and most supportive friendships seem to have been with women, and I would like to look at two women in particular who were important to her, Sophia Jex-Blake and Harriot Yorke.

Sophia Jex-Blake is most familiar today as one of the early women doctors, but her friendship with Octavia began some years before this stage of her life when she was employed as a mathematics tutor at Queens College, where Octavia's sister Emily was also a student. They got to know each other at the beginning of 1860 when Octavia began to give Sophia book-keeping lessons. In return Sophia taught Octavia maths – not a very romantic start, but the sense of excitement in this early getting-to-know-each-other stage is conveyed in their letters. I have recorded extracts from some of their letters and Sophia's diary entries[38] because they give the most vivid picture of their relationship, and how it deepened from initial liking and attraction into something much more significant. Octavia was 20 at this time and Sophia 18.

> Sophia (diary, 26 January 1860): Just had a lesson in book-keeping from Miss Hill. Clever pleasant girl – much nicer than I thought. Dined with me. . . .[39]

> Octavia (letter to Miranda and Florence, 5 February 1860): I've been giving some book-keeping lessons to Miss J.B. She is a bright, spirited, brave, generous young lady living alone in true bachelor style. It took me three nights to teach her and she begged me to to come to dinner each time. . . .[40]

Octavia (letter to Miranda, 29 April 1860): I'm as merry as a grig. . . . Miss J.B. and I are great companions. I'm always doing things with her. You know she's teaching me Euclid. We went to see Holman Hunt's picture. . . .[41]

Sophia (diary entry, undated, probably April 1860): My dear loving strong child [Octavia]. I do love and reverence her. . . . Had a loving solemn letter (not altogether pleasing to me on my telling her we had had a 'row') [at home]. Told her by return 'Hang you', and bade her to remember she was neither nurse nor parson. Dear, dear child, though.[42]

Sophia (diary 17 May 1860): Told Octa about Wales, – sitting in her room on the table, my heart beating like a hammer. That Carry wanted to go to Wales and I too, and most convenient about beginning of July, so . . . 'Put off my visit?' said Octa. 'No I was going to say (slowly) if you wish to see anything of me, you must come too, I think, and not put off the mountains until heaven.' She sunk her head on my lap silently, raised it in tears, and then such a kiss![43]

Sophia (letter to her mother, 30 July 1860): All over, darling, now, and such a happy time without a single blot I never remember in my life. Everything has been better than any anticipation of it. . . . Octavia looks five years younger, and as bright as a sunbeam. And I am in so thoroughly happy a state of mind as hardly to know myself. I really almost think that I should be good-tempered now. . . . I cannot say that I am glad that our tour is over, for I do believe that I was never so happy in my whole life . . .[44]

Octavia (letter to Sophia, August 1860): London feels strangely desolate, the lamps looked as they used to look, pityless and unending as I walked home last night, and knew I could not go to you. . . . I look forward to bright long days in which I shall learn always more about you, and watch with unending and unfathomable love and sympathy your upward growth, and we may look back together on our lives, as I do often on my own. . . .[45]

Sophia (diary, 9 September 1860): A plan on foot of my taking part in a house with the Hills. . . . That would be very jolly.[46]

Octavia (letter to Sophia, 18 October 1860): My Darling Child, Thanks for all the trouble that you are taking about the houses.

I am quite ashamed that it should all fall to your share. ...
Don't weary yourself with searching. I will certainly return on
Thursday (probably much before) then we will look together
again. ... I am writing in the dark. Goodbye, my own darling
treasure.[47]

Octavia (letter to Sophia, December 1860): Oh, child, your
letters are such a delight, but I miss you so dreadfully. I wander
about the house and long for you intensely. Every place seems
desolate. Your room, the fire, the thought of all you had told
me to provide for myself, fills my eyes with tears.[48]

Sophia and the Hills found a house together at 14 Nottingham
Place and in December 1860 Sophia moved in with Octavia and
her mother and sisters. In May of the following year Octavia was
called away to Cumberland to help a sick friend. In her absence
it appears that Sophia and Mrs Hill, Octavia's mother, did not
get on at all well together. There were a number of rows, and in
October Octavia was summoned home by her mother to deal with
the situation. We do not know what was said, but possibly Mrs
Hill presented Octavia with some sort of ultimatum, because after
their talk she asked Sophia to leave the house and changed the
nature of their relationship. They continued to see each other for
a while, and Octavia was to write Sophia a number of tender
letters over the next few years, but their intimacy was never
renewed. Sophia was utterly heartbroken as the next few extracts
show:

Sophia (diary, 13 December 1861): The loss of Octavia's day,
– her visit of one hour – the utter stupor of misery.[49]

Sophia (undated letter, probably to her mother, 1 December
1861): I am thinking how near 4 o'clock is coming. It may bring
me a kiss or a word from my darling. I'm sure tonight's post
will at any rate.[50]

Sophia (diary 31 December 1861): The last day of the year!
Now to 'take stock'. How well I remember last year. Does she?
How we did and sorted accounts till the chimes, – and then
leant together out of the window in our new house fresh with
plans and hopes, saying hopefully,
'*And may the New Year cherish,*
All the hopes that now are bright.'

And now truly almost, '*For all my earthly hopes this (year) did kill.*'[51]

Sophia (diary, 1862): But while I have at last manfully and honestly and cheerily faced the possibility of never seeing her again on earth ... yet it is curious how the whole fashion of my life shapes itself with the *arrière-pensée* of being ready for her 'at midnight or cock-crowing in the morning', saving with the thought of her as well as myself, – looking at every path as it opens to see that it is wide enough to tread together if she joins me ere its end. ...[52]

The relationship was over, finished by Octavia. She obviously still cared deeply for Sophia, and was grieved by the pain she was going through, but she never allowed their old intimacy to be renewed. Sophia found it impossible to let go of her hopes of a renewal of the relationship. For many years she made touching references to her in her diary – 'Octa always said',[53] 'How Octa'd laughed.'[54]

Sophia (diary, 28 March 1868): Is my old idea ever to work out by Octavia Hill studying medicine? *Wouldn't* she be a good doctor?[55]

Sophia (diary, May 1877, on hearing of Octavia's breach with John Ruskin): Oh dear! I'm ashamed of the first sort of thrill of triumph that she should know how it hurts.[56]

Sophia (diary April 1878): My life is full again if somewhat greyer for all the pain and, if I can have J [unidentified], the former things can abide in shadow till the day of restitution of all things. I can't but believe that some day, some where I shall learn what it all meant. ...[57]

These extracts will strike a chord with anyone who has ever been through an unhappy love affair, and I think that it can only be described as a love affair. The key question which emerges in deciding this, is whether continuity is a hallmark of friendship or not. All the rest of Octavia's major friendships seemed to last and to deepen over time. This one must have been different – it abruptly changed character – and this seems more characterisic of a love affair than a friendship. Significantly she never saw Edward Bond again either after their engagement was broken off.

After the break Sophia followed Octavia's life and work with unfailing interest; she subscribed to various of Octavia's schemes and in repeated wills she left her the whole of her property.[58] In 1910, when Octavia wrote her anti-suffrage letter to *The Times*, she too wrote to the paper regretting that Miss Hill should 'have given the support of her honoured name' to the negative side of the controversy[59] (the letter was not in fact published). She then wrote to Octavia, hoping that they could meet again to discuss the issue.

> I am rheumatic and lame now, and cannot go about much, but I wish you would come down and spend two or three days with me here on the Sussex hills, and we would thrash out this Suffrage question – surely one of us ought to be able to convince the other! And I *should* like to see you again![60]

This poignant appeal was written some fifty years after the end of their relationship, and in a romantic novel a reconciliation would have been made. Sadly, this was real life and no such happy ending materialised – Octavia replied to the letter, but she did not respond to Sophia's appeal that they meet again and two years later they both died.

We cannot be sure of the reasons why Octavia so resolutely changed the nature of her relationship with Sophia. On the surface it seems that she was bowing to family pressure, but possibly there were other factors. Sophia's diary refers to 'cataracts and breaks' on both sides, and there are letters of penitence for hot temper or 'coldness and pride'.[61] And for Octavia, emotional peace was very important. She wrote to Sophia in July 1861 when she had received another appeal to come home to sort out the discord there.

> I hold myself prepared to come when it seems right, sure to be given strength to do my duty, but certainly not longing for anything that will bring me again into a world of contention. ... All my life long this dreadful misery about even the slightest contention or estrangement has taken the form of misery, continually saying in itself 'I can*not* bear it'.[62]

It seems that for Octavia the cost of the sort of emotional upheaval that Sophia brought into her life outweighed the joy and excitement which she clearly got from the relationship. She survived the break-up better than Sophia. Sophia went on to do great work in opening up medical training for women and, by any standards, lived a rich and exciting life, but she never got over Octavia. 'She was never the same again,' said a life-long friend, 'it cut her life in two.'[63]

Margaret Todd's biography of Sophia, from which I have drawn most of these extracts, was published in 1918, and subsequent writers on both women have commented on the intense nature of their attachment.[64] I am not claiming to have uncovered a previously unknown facet of Octavia's life, but I do think it to be more than the adolescent episode or romantic friendship which some commentators take it to be. I am aware of the work that has been done on Victorian women's romantic friendships, and of the dangers of reading too much into them. Lillian Faderman, in her study of romantic friendships between women, says that '. . . it was virtually impossible to study the correspondence of any 19th century woman . . . and not uncover a passionate commitment to some other woman at some time in her life.'[65] Philippa Levine argues that:

> Such friendships were often intense and passionate, involving declarations of love and promises of eternity not dissimilar to those found in the language of romantic heterosexuality – the nineteenth century women's movement offers so many examples of deep and unashamed love between women – who often chose to spend their lives together – that the specifics of genital contact seem an irrelevant index of these friendships.[66]

I am not sure whether I want to speculate whether this was a lesbian relationship or not. It would be presumptuous and perhaps voyeuristic of me to make inferences about the sexual life and inclinations of two people who can in no sense give me permission to do so. It does raise the question of whether women can be lesbian in the physical sense if they have never heard of the concept and we do not know whether Octavia and Sophia had or not. It is also difficult to imagine the extremely pious Octavia engaging in anything even slightly improper. I am not so sure about Sophia. She wrote in her diary, 'I believe I love women too much ever to love a man. Yet who can tell. Well, SJB, don't get sentimental for pity's sake.' [67]

As Sheila Jeffreys[68] points out, however, the distinction between passionate friendships and lesbianism is, in fact, a very hard one to draw. Commenting on the intense friendships which existed between Victorian women she says: 'whether or not these women expressed themselves genitally there is no doubt that physical excitement and eroticism played an important part in their love',[69] and she cites Sophia's account of Octavia's kiss [she sunk her head on my lap silently, raised it in tears, and then such a kiss!] as an example of this, saying that it was no 'platonic peck on the cheek which is being described here'.[70] There was certainly nothing furtive though about Sophia's feelings for Octavia – she wrote about them freely to her mother – it was not 'a love that dare not speak its name'.

Significantly, though, the collections of Octavia's letters published by her family after her death, which celebrated the warmth and breadth of Octavia's friendships, contain none of the correspondence between Octavia and Sophia and no account of this important friendship, not even the fact that Sophia lived with the Hills for some nine months. Margaret Todd suggests that the extracts given in her biography of Sophia 'are a mere gleaning from many unpublished letters which bear witness to her [Octavia's] devoted attachment to SJB'.[71] Possibly the episode aroused memories which were still too painful to record, but it was an act of censorship which points to the fact that Octavia's family, for whatever reasons, did not wish this part of her life to be recorded for posterity.

I think that Sophia and Octavia were truly, deeply, madly in love, and that this was a relationship which transcended the boundaries of friendship. It also shows a side to Octavia which has been overlooked – her capacity both for this sort of passionate involvement with another woman, and her strength to renounce it when it got in the way of family duty and her work. She was devoted to her mother and sisters and had a very strong sense of family duty – and once duty had been decided upon it could not be turned back upon, no matter the personal cost. She wrote to her friend Mary Harris:

> How the real bond of family re-asserts itself, dominant over fancy, attraction, yes even perhaps, in a measure, over friendship itself! as though it would teach us how tremendous is the bond of duty. Certainly we have duties to our friends too; but they seem to have more relation to what we feel instinctive longing to do, innate capacity for doing, – to stand more by virtue of relations we have chosen for ourselves, than solely, wholly on the command of God.[72]

It also sheds light on some of the steel Octavia showed in housing management, her determination to evict those who would not pay the rent or who did not come up to her standards of housekeeping, no matter how piteous their appeals. One of her first acts on taking over her first housing scheme in Paradise Place was to evict a widow and her four children, although she said her heart was wrung by their plight:

> if thou couldst have seen the drunken widow, who awaited me at the door, her four children, ragged and miserable, entreating to be taken back into the house which she had kept in that state, and how the hope died out of her eyes as she saw all the men of business with me, and how she fell back without even uttering the request she had made in the morning. I was so weary and sick at heart. . . .[73]

Octavia went on to have other very close relationships with women, but perhaps none as intense as that with Sophia. She was clearly very fond of Jane Nassau Senior (the sister of Thomas Hughes) who helped out with the accounts in Octavia's early housing schemes. It was Octavia who persuaded Lord Stansfield, a COS colleague and President of the Local Government Board, to appoint Jane Nassau Senior as first woman poor law inspector of workhouses (a nice example of women's networking?). She addressed her in her letters as 'dearest Janey' and wrote on her death in 1877:

> she loved me, as few do; and I her; and, when I think that I can go to her no more, I dare not think what the loss will be . . . the thought that I can never again in human word receive any message from her shakes me with passionate sobbing. . . .[74]

In 1877, at the age of 39, Octavia met the woman who was to become her life-long companion – Miss Harriot Yorke. Harriot Yorke is something of a shadowy figure. She first emerges as travelling companion for Octavia when she went abroad to recover from a collapse in mental and physical health in 1878 following a series of calamitous events – the deaths of her friends Jane Nassau Senior and Sidney Cockerell, a rift with Ruskin, and the breaking off of her engagement to Edward Bond. They established a very close relationship and in 1884, when the school which Octavia's sisters ran in their house finally closed, Harriot moved in with the family. She also helped with the housing work, and as a woman of means bought property for Octavia's housing schemes and a country cottage for them both at Crockham Hill, near Octavia's sister Gertrude's country home.[75] Harriot later became treasurer of the National Trust. Something of the flavour of their relationship is conveyed by their nicknames for each other – Octavia was known as the 'Lion' and Harriot the 'Keeper'.[76] She seems to have been a stabilising factor in Octavia's life. Up to this point she had suffered a series of emotional and physical crises necessitating long periods of recovery, but after she met Harriot these ceased.[77] Moberley Bell, in her biography of Octavia, claims that 'she had never been looked after before. She found it wonderfully pleasant'.[78] Unlike Sophia, Harriot was accepted by Mrs Hill, and there seem to have been no family rifts over this friendship. Moberley Bell comments of the relationship: 'Thence arose a satisfying friendship which became the most precious possession of them both. It was such a relationship as is supposed to be peculiarly characteristic of English spinsters.'[79] Again it is difficult to know the exact nature of this relationship, but it does seem to point once more to the fact that Octavia's emotional point of reference was women.

Sisters also performed an important role. Octavia had close relationships with all her sisters – Miranda, Emily, Gertrude and Florence – all of whom worked with her in her housing schemes at various times. In 1878 when illness forced her to take her long holiday abroad, her sisters, friends and fellow workers took over all her responsibilities. Octavia wrote to her mother from abroad:

> My thoughts of you all make me realise how you are all doing, and have done so much, ... How I think of you all, of dear Andy [Miranda] bearing the burden of all management; of dear Florence keeping to work with her frail health; of dear Gertrude so marvellously carrying on my work; and of dear Minnie [Emily] doing all so perfectly and thinking of everyone.[80]

She was particularly close to her eldest sister Miranda, who lived with her all her adult life. She was a mainstay to her in her work and a great emotional support. Miranda, although active in her own right – founding the Kyrle Society (an organisation aimed at 'the diffusion of art in the life of the people') and becoming a poor law guardian – played a very much secondary and supportive role to Octavia, and seemed to have been glad to do so. She wrote to a friend in 1884: 'Octavia's work is so wide and many-sided, and she is so large-hearted and wise in giving all her fellow-workers leave to work in their own way, that she often hands a little domain over to me to work in my own way.'[81] Miranda also seemed to provide domestic support, and to play a nurturing role to this dominant sister. 'It feels like home now Miranda is back again,' Octavia wrote to her mother in 1889, 'and it is wonderful to see the atmosphere of love and peace she spreads around her.'[82] And Octavia performed the masculine role of head of household, though why this should have been when she was not even the oldest sister is not quite clear. It was she who handled the family finances and who was responsible for getting lodgings and paying off family debts. While she accepted this duty, she says feelingly at one point that her family seemed to think her 'good only to do a sum, carry a weight, go a long walk in the rain, or decide any difficult question about tangible things'.[83]

This supportive sisterly role also comes across strongly in Emma Cons' relationship with her sister Ellen. Emma Cons was one of Octavia's oldest friends and the first of her paid workers, and she became a large-scale housing worker in her own right. She lived in at Surrey Buildings, one of the housing schemes which she ran, together with two sisters Ellen and Elisa, and a friend, Caroline Martineau, who acted as her secretary. Her niece Lilian Baylis also moved in with her aunts when she came back from South Africa. Emma then, like Octavia, chose to live with sisters and friends and, like Octavia, she enjoyed close and supportive relationships with her sisters. Emma and Ellen had a particularly close relationship. Their niece Lilian Baylis wrote:

> My aunt Ellen was perhaps the most invaluable to Emmie's work; we used to say that Emmie was like the strong husband and Ellen the devoted wife. Whatever time Emmie came home from her work, there was always every comfort awaiting her; and whatever difficulties had arisen during her absence – over the housing or over the Vic – Ellen had dealt with, to the best of her power and ability. Emmie, I am certain, could never have accomplished the half of what she did, without Ellen's loving care at home.[84]

Emma's reliance on her sister Ellen is striking and bears a strong resemblance to Octavia's dependence on her sister Miranda. Possibly the difficulties of making a career and running a home would have been too great at this time to have been undertaken without this sort of almost 'wifely' support at home. It is certainly difficult to imagine a man, especially a Victorian man – either husband or brother – providing this kind of support, and being content with playing an invisible background role.

It is interesting too that Emma is characterised as the 'strong husband', Octavia notes in her letters that when her sisters want to refer to her as their brother they called her Loke; '"Loke" is my name with which is associated all my strength; it is Florence's own invention, whenever my sisters call me their brother, then I am "Loke".'[85] Florence Hill wrote to her sister Emily in 1866 that 'Ockey is rather like a *man* taking a holiday; she thinks it her duty to be idle, and does not know quite what to do with herself . . .'.[86] Given the strong emphasis, in Octavia's writings at least, on womanly duties and virtues, one wonders what sort of unconscious role-playing was going on here.

Other workers also lived in the households of Octavia and Emma Cons from time to time, and this intermingling of home and work life seems to have been one of the most distinctive features of single women's involvement in social work at this period. Certainly it is not a feature of women social workers' lives today who would not expect to have to live with their employers. Living-in may have had something to do with the difficulty that single women experienced in finding suitable and congenial accommodation. Possibly anxious parents would have expressed less opposition to their daughters' plans to leave home and work in housing schemes in rough areas if they were reassured that they would be living in respectable and supervised households. It may also have been less daunting to the women in launching themselves into a new path in life to live among like-minded friends. Whatever the factors involved, such intimate living and working arrangements must have made for very much closer relationships between Octavia and Emma and their workers than those which normally exist between colleagues. It must also have bonded together fellow workers into a definite community with close personal as well as professional ties. Perhaps in forging new careers in the public world as these women were, this feeling of mutual support reinforced a sense of the correctness of their chosen course and acted as some sort of protection against the opposition which they undoubtedly faced. It may also have been possible that they were carrying over their normal way of operating into their new roles. Middle-class Victorian women did, after all, spend a good deal of their time staying with each other and going on holiday together and this intermingling of work and social life may have been a feature of the first generation of middle-class women moving into the new world of work. Certainly work is a much more separate activity for us now, but for nineteenth-century middle-class women paid work was a new experience and they had no idea of its conventions. And this sense of the alien nature of the male world of work carried over well into the twentieth century. Jill Tweedie, the feminist journalist, writing of her introduction to the world of work in the 1960s says:

> For me the working world was another country. . . . My father, and all the men in my childhood and adolescence, daily travelled in and out but appeared to be bound by some Mafia oath never to talk of what happened there to wives, daughters or anyone else of the female sex. . . . I remained, as ever, unable to discern the divisions between public and private, contacts and friends, kindness and more venal favours, the business world and the personal; it was all one to me.[87]

The divisions between public and private were just as unclear to these early women workers and they brought their normal way of relating to their friends into the world of work. Henrietta Barnett says that her group of workers used to meet with her and her husband once a week: 'not only to talk over the people under their care, but to get to know and thereby sustain each other. What fun we used to have amid all the difficulties!'[88] Miss Townsend, one of Henrietta's workers, gives the same impression of the joys of shared work:

> very soon a group of ladies, young and ardent, gathered around us, each as the years went on caring for a number of poor girls to whom she was guide, example and support. Ah! what good times they are to look back upon, when day by day in our little room at 28 Commercial Street, our own girls came to us confident that we would help them on their steep and often erring way. Those of who have lived to grow old together have a bond of union nothing could ever break.[89]

This is a very vivid evocation of the sort of comradeship, loyalty and affection that was engendered among women working in a common cause. It is echoed in the accounts of many of the women activists of the time and Annie Kenney, one of the leading members of the Women's Social and Political Union, said of her time in the suffragette movement that 'No companionship can ever surpass the companionship of the militants during the childhood and youth of the suffragette fight.'[90]

All of Octavia's workers were women as she insisted that housing management was solely a female profession. In the early days her workers were drawn from her circle of friends and acquaintances, but as the work grew they came to her from all over the country, and indeed the world. She was extremely successful in attracting other women to work with her, and her sister Miranda nicknamed her St Ursula because of her capacity for attracting disciples and followers.[91] And clearly her fellow workers were of great importance to Octavia. She wrote in 1877: 'It is well for me that in the course of work I do naturally see many of my friends; and that I do love and care very deeply for many of my fellow workers.'[92] A key feature of Octavia's work was the trust she placed in her fellow workers. The work did not depend on her alone, and she urged her workers to work as independently of her as possible and devolved responsibility wherever she could. 'My ideal', she said, ' is the utmost possible independence of the lady in charge of the houses.'[93] She encouraged and supported her fellow workers, and above all had a great feeling of shared endeavour with them. This must have done a great deal to encourage these women's confidence in stepping into the public world of employment for the first time. Many of Octavia's workers went on to other public positions. Henrietta Barnett was made a Dame of the British Empire in recognition of her service to the community, Emma Cons was the first woman to be made an alderman of London County Council, and Beatrice Webb, the best known of these early women housing workers, went on to an outstanding public career.

This emphasis on warm personal relationships between workers also spills over into work with tenants. One of the guiding principles of Octavia's work in housing was that it should be done on an individual basis and that her tenants were individually known – 'For, firstly my people are numbered; not merely counted, but known, man, woman and child,'[94] she argued, 'Think what this mere fact of being known is to the poor.'[95] She did not believe that any impersonal society or organisation could work effectively with the tenants: 'there needs, and will need for some time, a reformatory work which will demand that loving zeal of individuals which cannot be had for money, and cannot be legislated for by Parliament.'[96] She also had very strong, almost maternal feelings about her tenants, declaring in a letter to a friend in 1869, 'But my people, oh, my people, how I love them more and more.'[97]

And while she worked for working-class families, not women as such, it was with the women tenants she had most contact. Housing work enabled women to work with other women and, on the whole, for women. Octavia did not talk of her work in terms of a women's mission to women, but by its very nature it impinged most directly on women. Like social work today, it was aimed at the most poor and powerless in society, and then as now these were predominantly women. In both housing and the relief work with which Octavia was involved, the dealings of the workers were almost exclusively with women. In one of her essays on the distribution of relief, Octavia comments:

> The application for help is nearly always made by the wife, and the respectable husband would no more make it than you or I would, in nine cases out of ten. Only notice what happens whenever the rule is that the man must come up to ask for help; they hardly ever come, but simply earn the needed amount.[98]

It was women who bore the brunt of the poverty and faced the daily struggle of feeding their families, and is not surprising that they should be the ones who swallowed their pride and faced up to the humiliating task of applying for relief. (See also Chapter 3.) Octavia recognised the hardness of the lot of her women tenants and she wrote to a friend:

> Such worn, haggard and careworn women cringing down to me, who has never suffered and struggled as they have without teaching or help, deadened to all sense of order or cleanliness and self-respect. 'My friends', I feel inclined to say to them, 'don't treat me with such respect. In spirit I bow down to you, feeling that you deserve reverence, in that you have preserved any atom of God's image in you, degraded and battered as you are by the world's pressure.'[99]

One cannot overlook the class dimension to Octavia's work nor the element of control it involved, but to me what comes over from this passage is a sense not only of respect for, and empathy with, her poor women tenants, but an extension of Octavia's feelings for women in all aspects of her life. She loved her fellow workers, she loved her tenants and she certainly seems to have loved her women friends. Relationships motivated Octavia in her work as much as in her private life, and I do not think that the two can be separated. She wrote to her sister Emily in 1856:

> I intend to accept no work however delightful, however remumerative (except as a temporary thing), which would deprive me of the power of working for others. . . . That which I *do* care for is the intercourse, sympathy, self-sacrifice, and mutual help which are called out in fellow workers; and this I believe to be worth striving for; this I mean to work for.[100]

This was written before she had begun her career in housing and it sets the tone for the rest of her life and work; the personal and the private cannot be separated from the political and the public.

NOTES

1 Foreword to E. Moberley Bell, *Octavia Hill: a Biography*, London, Constable, 1942, p. ix.
2 See Gillian Darley, *Octavia Hill: A Life*, London, Constable, 1990, p. 29.
3 N. G. Annan, 'The Intellectual Aristocracy', in J. H. Plumb (ed.), *Studies in Social History*, Longman, Green, 1955.
4 Jane Rendall (ed.), *Equal or Different: Women's Politics 1800–1914*, Oxford, Basil Blackwell, 1987, p. 10.
5 Ray Strachey, *The Cause: A Short History of the Women's Movement in Great Britain*, G. Bell & Sons, 1928.
6 Martha Vicinus, *Independent Women: Work and Community for Single Women 1850–1920*, London, Virago Press, 1985, p. 30.
7 Liz Stanley, *Feminism and Friendship: Two Essays on Olive Schreiner*, Studies in Sexual Politics, No. 8, Department of Sociology, University of Manchester, 1985.
8 Ibid., p. 3.
9 Philippa Levine, *Feminist Lives in Victorian England: Private Lives and Public Commitment*, Oxford, Basil Blackwell, 1990.
10 Ibid., p. 10.
11 See the selection of letters between Ruskin and Octavia Hill in Emily S. Maurice (ed.), *Octavia Hill: Early Ideals*, London, George Allen & Unwin, 1928.
12 Gareth Stedman-Jones states that 22,466 persons, mainly casual persons, were displaced by the Artisans' Dwellings Acts between 1883

and 1895, see Gareth Stedman-Jones, *Outcast London: A Study in the Relationship between Classes in Victorian Society*, Penguin Books, 1984, p. 326.

13 Octavia Hill, 'Landlords and Tenants in London', in *Homes of the London Poor*, London, Macmillan, 1875, pp. 102–3.

14 E. S. Ouvry (ed.), *Octavia Hill's Letters on Housing, 1864–1911*, London, The Adelphi Bookshop, 1933, p. 23.

15 Ibid., p. 13.

16 Ibid., p. 47.

17 Society of Women Housing Managers, *Housing Estate Management* (being an account of the development of the work initiated by Octavia Hill), 1946, p. 2.

18 See Darley, *Octavia Hill: A Life*, p. 256.

19 See Moberley Bell, *Octavia Hill: A Biography*, p. 277.

20 Jane Lewis, *Women and Social Action in Victorian and Edwardian England*, Cheltenham, Edward Elgar Publishing, 1991, p. 26.

21 E. Moberley Bell, *Octavia Hill: A Biography*, p. 270.

22 Quoted in Darley, *Octavia Hill: A Life*, p. 319.

23 Miranda Hill to Mary Harris, in Moberley Bell, *Octavia Hill: A Biography*, p. 240.

24 E. Moberley Bell, *Octavia Hill: A Biography*, p. 270.

25 Octavia Hill, 'District Visiting', in *Our Common Land*, London, Macmillan, 1877, pp. 24–5.

26 See Octavia Hill to Miss Baumgartner, 22 December 1863, in C. E. Maurice, *Life of Octavia Hill as Told in Her Letters*, London, Macmillan, 1913, p. 208.

27 See Octavia Hill to Miss Davies, 18 February 1864, in C. E. Maurice, *Life of Octavia Hill*, pp. 209–10.

28 See Darley, *Octavia Hill: A Life*, p. 137.

29 Ibid.

30 Stanley, *Feminism and Friendship*, p. 21.

31 Parliamentary Papers 1884–85, Royal Commission on the Housing of the Working Classes, 8964.

32 C. E. Maurice, *Life of Octavia Hill*, p. 582.

33 Marion Brion and Anthea Tinker, *Women in Housing: Access and Influence*, London, Housing Centre Trust, 1980, p. 71.

34 Henrietta Barnett, *Canon Barnett: His Life, Work and Friends*, London, John Murray, 1921, p. 106.

35 See Elizabeth Sturge, *Reminiscences of my Life, and Some Account of the Children of William and Charlotte Sturge and of the Sturge Family of Bristol*, printed for private circulation, Bristol, 1928.

36 Octavia Hill to Miss Florence Davenport Hill, 9 June 1869, in C. E. Maurice, *Life of Octavia Hill*, p. 254.

37 See C. E. Maurice, *Life of Octavia Hill*, p. 261.

38 Sophia Jex-Blake's diary entries and letters, and some of Octavia Hill's letters, are taken from Margaret Todd, *The Life of Sophia Jex-Blake*, London, Macmillan, 1918. The other letters from Octavia Hill are taken from C. E. Maurice, *Life of Octavia Hill*.

39 Margaret Todd, *The Life of Sophia Jex-Blake*, p. 84.

40 C. E. Maurice, *Life of Octavia Hill*, p. 177.
41 Ibid., p. 180.
42 Margaret Todd, *The Life of Sophia Jex-Blake*, p. 85.
43 Ibid., pp. 85–6.
44 Ibid., p. 86.
45 Ibid., p. 87.
46 Ibid., p. 88.
47 Ibid., p. 89.
48 Ibid., pp. 89–90.
49 Ibid., p. 96.
50 Ibid., p. 97.
51 Ibid., pp. 100–1.
52 Ibid., p. 116.
53 Ibid., p. 109.
54 Ibid., p. 110.
55 Ibid., p. 199.
56 Ibid., p. 468.
57 Ibid., p. 468.
58 Ibid., p. 94.
59 Ibid., p. 538.
60 Ibid., p. 538.
61 Ibid., p. 88.
62 Ibid., p. 90.
63 Ibid., p. 95.
64 See, e.g., E. Moberley Bell, 1942; Josephine Kamm, 1966; Philippa
    Levine, 1990; Gillian Darley, 1990.
65 Lillian Faderman, *Surpassing the Love of Men: Romantic Friendship
    and Love between Women from the Renaissance to the Present*, The
    Women's Press, 1985, p. 16.
66 Levine, *Feminist Lives*, p. 68.
67 Todd, *The Life of Sophia Jex-Blake*, p. 65.
68 Sheila Jeffreys, *The Spinster and her Enemies: Feminism and Sexuality
    1880–1930*, London, Pandora Press, 1985.
69 Ibid., p. 104.
70 Ibid.
71 Todd, *The Life of Sophia Jex-Blake*, p. 92.
72 Octavia Hill to Miss Harris, October or November, 1860, in C. E.
    Maurice, *The Life of Octavia Hill*, pp. 185–6.
73 Letter to Mary Harris, no date, probably 1864, in E. S. Maurice,
    Octavia Hill: Early Ideals, p. 191.
74 Octavia to Sydney Cockerell, 21 March 1877, in C. E. Maurice, *Life
    of Octavia Hill*, p. 349.
75 Moberley Bell, *Octavia Hill: A Biography*, p. 181.
76 Ibid., p. 166.
77 I am indebted for this insight to Theresa Deane.
78 Moberley Bell, *Octavia Hill: A Biography*, p. 165.
79 Ibid., pp. 165–6.
80 Octavia Hill to her mother, 14 March 1878, in C. E. Maurice, *Life of
    Octavia Hill*, p. 363.

81 Miranda Hill to Miss Durrant, 12 December 1890, in C. E. Maurice, *Life of Octavia Hill*, p. 515.

82 Octavia Hill to her mother, 28 April 1889, in C. E. Maurice, *Life of Octavia Hill*, p. 501.

83 Octavia Hill to John Ruskin, February 1859, cited in C. E. Maurice, *Life of Octavia Hill*, p. 131.

84 Cicely Hamilton and Lilian Baylis, *The Old Vic*, London, Jonathan Cape, 1926, p. 256.

85 Octavia Hill to Miss Harrison, 1 August 1855, quoted in C. E. Maurice, *Life of Octavia Hill*, p. 55.

86 Florence Hill to Emily Hill, 29 July 1866, in C. E. Maurice, *Life of Octavia Hill*, p. 224.

87 Jill Tweedie, *Eating Children*, with an unfinished memoir, Frightening People, Penguin Books, 1994, pp. 350–2.

88 Barnett, *Canon Barnett*, p. 133.

89 Ibid., p. 120.

90 Annie Kenney, *Memories of a Militant*, London, Edward Arnold, 1924.

91 C. E. Maurice, *Life of Octavia Hill*, p. 240.

92 Octavia to Mrs Gillum, 7 February 1877, in C. E. Maurice, *Life of Octavia Hill*, p. 347.

93 Ouvry, *Octavia Hill's Letters on Housing*, p. 13.

94 Octavia Hill, 'Management of a London Court', in *Homes of the London Poor*, London, Macmillan, 1875, p. 57.

95 Ibid., p. 60.

96 Octavia Hill, Preface to *Homes of the London Poor*, p. 7.

97 Octavia to Mary Harris, 11 July 1869 in E. S. Maurice, *Octavia Hill: Early Ideals*, p. 105.

98 Octavia Hill, 'A More Excellent Way of Charity', in *Our Common Land*, p. 84.

99 Octavia to Mary Harris, no date (probably 1864), in E. S. Maurice, *Octavia Hill: Early Ideals*, p. 190.

100 Octavia Hill to Emily Hill, 18 February 1856, in C. E. Maurice, *Life of Octavia Hill*, p. 74.

Chapter 5

Late nineteenth-century philanthropy
The case of Louisa Twining[1]

Theresa Deane

Modern scholarship generally makes passing reference to Louisa Twining either in the context of philanthropy, the poor law, workhouse nursing or women's history with the focus on the changing public and private lives of middle- and upper-class women. In all of these she is associated with health or welfare.[2] However, Twining has not been studied in any depth and there is only a single article solely devoted to her life and work.[3] This chapter is part of an attempt to retrieve and examine her life comprehensively, with the focus on her so-called retirement years. It is assumed that Twining's work was serious, and that its progress and development can be described as a career. Although it is not unusual to analyse philanthropic work by concentrating on individuals, this chapter aims to break new ground by examining philanthropy as employment.[4]

Louisa Twining was born in 1820 and grew up in London only a short distance from where her father worked, in the tea and coffee business established by her great-great-grandfather Thomas Twining.[5] She was the youngest by five years of the eight surviving children of Richard and Elizabeth Twining. Louisa was taught skills such as reading, writing and needlework by her elder sister Elizabeth, who had in her turn been taught by their mother, as was conventional within their circle of friends.[6] She acquired the necessary accomplishments for an upper middle-class woman through painting lessons, which she enjoyed, and piano lessons, which she did not. This was augmented by classes in several languages taught by a variety of masters. Louisa also attended lectures at the Royal Institution. She considered these the most important part of her education, and continued to attend public lectures into her twenties.[7] Her liberal education

was completed by foreign tours, and she never lost her love of
travelling.

During her twenties she attended bible classes given by the
Christian Socialist, Frederick Maurice, in his home, as well as
attending a course of his lectures on moral philosophy at his
newly opened Queen's College.[8] Her brothers – William, Aldred
and Richard – were, typically, more advantaged. They attended
Thomas Arnold's Rugby, all three went to Oxford before pursuing
careers in, respectively, medicine, the law and the family business
which by then included Twining's bank.[9]

The family's philanthropic activities were focused on their local
parish. All were practising members of the Church of England,
worshipping at St Clement Danes in the Strand. Her father,
and later her eldest brother, were, for example, treasurers for
the public dispensary in Carey Street, and her father was on the
Committee of Management of King's College Hospital, then in
Portugal Street, and on the vestry of St Clement Danes. Louisa's
sister Elizabeth, fifteen years her elder, was a district visitor,
taught in Sunday schools, was on the ladies committee of Queen's
College, and is credited with founding the Mother's Meeting
movement.[10]

In 1848 Louisa's brothers Aldred and William died within six
months of each other. She remembered this as a time of 'heavy
losses and trials' within her family circle and suggests that,
possibly, her 'attention was called to the condition of the poor'
because of these events.[11] Given her class, childhood, and culture
it is not surprising that the young Louisa Twining should undertake some philanthropic work.[12] What could not be predicted was
that she would devote her life to it.

Twining was Lady Superintendent of two Homes during her
forties and fifties. The first was the Workhouse Visiting Society's
Industrial Home. This trained workhouse girls for domestic service
and later expanded to provide care for elderly infirm women who
were looked after by some of the workhouse girls. The second
was St Luke's Home for Epileptic and Incurable Women which
was also a base for some nurse training and towards the end of
Twining's management offered accommodation to female art
students. In this way Twining, a single woman, created her own
home and family through her work, as a manager and provider
of welfare, by living in an all-female community. She was certainly
aware of the duality of public and private life even if she did not

have to reconcile the conflict of a public working life with that of a husband and children.

As well as managing these homes Twining was an active campaigner for the Workhouse Visiting Society (WVS) of which she was not only secretary but also editor of its journal.[13] Her public recognition was established in 1861 when she was invited to give evidence to the Select Committee on the Administration and Relief of the Poor. Here she expressed the need for improved nursing in workhouses, women inspectors, and women as poor law guardians.[14] She also published books and pamphlets linked to her work.

In 1882, aged almost 62, single and with no dependants, Louisa Twining decided to retire. She put her furniture in store, gave her pictures to worthy institutions and took a year-long holiday abroad. On her return she lived in Kensington where she served as a poor law guardian. She then briefly lived in Worthing where she set up a district nursing service before moving again, this time to Tunbridge Wells where she had spent childhood holidays, and served once more as a guardian. Twining campaigned for the Women's Guardians Society (WGS), was president and then vice-president of the Women in Local Government Society (WLGS), and was secretary, and later vice-president, of the Workhouse Nursing Association (WNA).[15] In her spare time she wrote two books of memoirs and at least twenty-five pamphlets besides having letters published regularly in various journals and the national press. What follows is an examination of the last three decades of her life until her death in 1912.

PHILANTHROPY

At its broadest, philanthropy is defined as 'an action or inclination which promotes the well-being of others'. This implies a personal relationship between donor and recipient, and is wide enough to include spontaneous actions – the stuff of casual benevolence among families and within neighbourhoods.[16] This is very much the way in which Twining began her philanthropic work in the 1840s as a visitor of the poor in the London parish of St Clement Danes. An alternative definition suggests that a necessary condition of philanthropy is 'the active promotion of "causes"'.[17] This is applicable to Twining's public work from March 1853 when she wrote to the Strand Board of Guardians

asking if she and two or three ladies could 'form a class for instruction, amongst the female inmates'.[18] Here is not only the sense
of benevolence (the promotion of welfare), but also a clear
objective in which a self-identified group of donors aims to reach
a specific recipient group. Twining's definition of recipients
developed from this limited one of able-bodied women in the
Strand Union into her first cause: the welfare of women, children,
the sick and the elderly among the indoor poor.

Philanthropy is also defined as a personal act and Twining's
Christian beliefs provided the explicit motivation for and justification of her work. Philanthropic work was her duty, and the duty
in this context was work which could be carried out in the public
realm of poor law administration. The following passage suggests
that she also saw the work as heaven-sent. Recalling the time
when she had just moved to Kensington she wrote:

> I soon began to wonder what I should find to occupy my time
> and thoughts, as I was not yet quite prepared for a life of leisure
> and idleness . . . so I waited to see what might come or be sent
> for me to do.[19]

Religion was also Twining's source of spiritual replenishment. She
kept it much more private at the end of her life while still using
its language. The Worthing District Nursing Committee was
'sanctioned' by eighteen men, ten of whom were clergymen.
Nursing was a 'happy and sacred calling', 'an arduous and responsible calling' and women's share in 'the social work' was part of
the 'Divine Order'.

Twining also used her religious belief to support the argument
that her work should be unpaid. Twining defined charity, which
she used as a synonym for almsgiving, as 'fervent, unselfish love'.[20]
It was a gift of money, time, skill or experience, and the cause
defined who were to be the recipients. If the donors were to be
rewarded it would be in the next world, not this: 'almsgiving' she
said, 'looks for nothing in return'.[21] Just as Twining did not require
a material return for almsgiving so she did not expect payment
for her work. The post of guardian was unpaid and therefore met
this important criterion. To be a guardian of the poor carried with
it the notion of *pro bono publico*, 'for the public good'. To be a
guardian was to be a public servant and no financial reward was
expected. This conveniently rebuffed any potential objections to
a woman born into the upper middle class who wished to work.

Twining always worked unpaid, with the exception of income from her writing. For a woman to earn money from writing, particularly on the subject of social problems, was well within the conventions of the time.

All of this obscures the non-financial benefits of philanthropy to Twining and women like her. She did not suggest that there was any personal gain from philanthropic work. Instead she turned the benefits of a full working life, the skills acquired and the career (with its full sense of ascendancy rather than just a sequence of posts) which women like her gained through their philanthropic welfare work, into her second cause: that of work for women. The cause of the welfare within the poor law of women, children and the sick fed the cause of women's work for, argued Twining, only women could provide for the welfare of their own sex, children, the elderly and the sick. The two causes were so closely integrated that it is difficult, perhaps conveniently for Twining, to separate them.

SELECTION, TRAINING AND ORGANISATIONAL STRUCTURES

Twining compared the workhouse to a domestic household, where it was recognised that women 'should have a place and a power of control'.[22] By doing so she secured a place for women in the management of the poor law. After all, she wrote, with 'four-fifths of our pauper population consisting of women and children, we do not consider it unreasonable that women should claim some responsibility in their management'.[23] The workhouses were public households and yet they were supervised by male guardians. She was surprised that

> so many womanly duties should hitherto have been performed by men alone – duties which we have no hesitation in saying would be scorned by them were they asked even to give an opinion upon them in their own households.[24]

Male inspectors were not safe from Twining's pen either. She said of her experiences of them that: 'Then as now, clever and highly educated gentlemen visited from time to time . . . as we suppose with the view of discovering defects.'[25]

As women managed the household, she wrote, so only women could regulate the domestic aspects of workhouses, such as inspecting the laundry, supervising the staff and monitoring the food. Twining used the model of domesticity not only to expose men's inability to regulate the operations of the workhouse but also to create a space for women's work as providers and managers. She saw no barrier to middle- and upper-class women having an active and independent public life, and challenged the prevailing idea that they had ever been confined to the home.

> The generation which is generally known as that of our grand-mothers, is considered to have been occupied by domestic and household work, and in the care of the family; but we are inclined to ask, if there was ever a time in which women were thus exclusively engaged?[26]

Twining therefore felt that women did not need to break into public life as they had never been confined to the domestic sphere, even if she had to draw her readers' attention to it. In the same article she urged women to take advantage of 'spheres of opportunities' already open to them, in particular as guardians of the poor. (See also Chapter 3.)

The use of gender as a means of defining work for men and work for women did not mean that the sexes were to operate in isolation. Twining wrote of disliking any single sex committee while simultaneously arguing that men and women had their own provinces. She justified this prescription for an integrated and yet separate male and female workforce by regular reference to Anna Jameson's *Communion of Labour*.[27] She used the concept to give approval and encouragement to women as they tried to secure their official place in public. Twining also used Jameson's philosophy to argue that the deficiencies of the workhouse and its inhuman care were caused by the lack of an integrated male and female management. Hence the feminine element of 'motherly and sisterly influence' was inadequately represented by the untrained workhouse matron and her pauper nurses.[28] Twining believed that women and men had different talents to offer, and that their roles were complementary.

Twining's vision of women's work became more precise as she moved from writing texts which predominantly justified the need for women's presence in the poor law to those which argued for women to be in specific posts: for example on hospital boards, as doctors, or working in other institutions such as lunatic asylums and prisons. She recorded the success of a woman who acted as relieving officer on behalf of her sick husband. In time she was appointed in her own right, because 'she was so perfectly efficient as his substitute'.[29] Twining's suggestions were permissive rather than directive and she was keenly aware of the difference.[30]

Her criteria for selection for occupations were negative as well as positive. She emphasised that nurses should be physically fit (thus excluding the elderly); educated (no matter what their social class); women of 'virtue' (in contrast to unmarried mothers); and women of judgement (unlike the workhouse matron). She used the word 'superior' – with all its connotations of class and respectability – to assign a status for women equal to that of professional for men. She was concerned that so many small tradesmen were being elected as guardians. This was due in part to the changing housing patterns in inner-city vestries such as St Clement Danes which the wealthy had forsaken for more salubrious areas as towns and cities expanded. Indeed Twining's own parents had moved to Bloomsbury in the mid-1830s.

Although guardians stood for election they were not always opposed. Twining was invited by a retiring guardian in Kensington to take his place, and in Tunbridge Wells she filled a vacancy caused by the death of the incumbent. She justified these actions by suggesting that they were an 'unsought-for opening' and 'the opening for work which I could not refuse'.[31] Her words convey a sense of mission and cause, combining both the spiritual and secular principles which motivated her work.

Twining was concerned that many suitable women were disbarred from being a Poor Law Guardian because of the property qualification for this office, and she argued for its reduction. She continued to support the post of ex-officio guardian (guardians co-opted by the elected guardians) until it was abolished in 1894. This was in spite of the fact, as she wryly pointed out, that ex-officio guardians were never women. Her recommendation for their continuance was part of her strategy to raise the quality of the guardians themselves. This way she believed 'superior' and educated people could be encouraged to work within the poor law. The argument for abolishing the ex-officio was that many were time-wasters, mere cronies of the elected men. However, Twining was not above wanting to recruit cronies from her female network who would not have been time-wasters. Despite this inconsistency, she argued for 'a competitive examination' for aspirant guardians in 'the spirit of the time'.[32]

Twining's desire for registration of poor law nurses was in part linked to her goal of objective recruitment. She saw it not only as an essential part of securing a poor law nursing profession but also as a way of doing away with testimonials in general which she described as 'examples of perfection', a good reference being an effective way of getting rid of unwanted staff by concealing their shortcomings.

Having selected the most suitable candidates Twining then wanted them trained, something she thought necessary 'for all professional work'.[33] She advocated training for guardians, nurses and even district visitors. She specified training goals rather than the training itself. Workhouse nurse training, for example, was to be nationally standardised, to result in a certificate, and to be distinct from training for nurses in voluntary hospitals.[34] Workhouse staff and guardians resisted the concept of nurse training because they did not want to lose control of the pauper nurse, and they feared that a professional nurse would introduce new practices and be less easy to manipulate.

Aware of inter-occupational conflicts, Twining sought to protect her trained nursing staff by the creation of a nursing management tree similar to that used by general nurses. There were tensions when trained nurses were accountable to the workhouse matron and master, with the result that there were even times when the master accompanied the doctor on his round and not the nurse. Twining's hierarchy consisted solely of trained nurses. Where three nurses were employed there was to be a superintendent, with overall responsibility being held by a matron. As ever, Twining used gender to argue that a woman with a nursing qualification was needed as an inspector in the Local Government Board: 'for gentlemen without medical training to examine into the state of the sick in infirmaries is preposterous and unreasonable'.[35] It was also quite unsuitable for the women to have to ask the male medical officer, who was usually just qualified and therefore young, about leave entitlement and the reasons for it.

In the workhouse nurses also needed the support of women guardians. Only women would think of asking about bed sores, or the inmates' food, or visiting the nurses at their meal times to see what food they were being given. Women as managers of domestic households, she argued, were accustomed to taking responsibility for staff welfare. Further, the women guardians were needed to deal with women's issues in general.[36] Twining was of necessity self-selected and untrained, and realised that she relied on her personal experience. However, she wanted a different future for her successors. She did not want to perpetuate the frustrations and the weakness of the unofficial worker who might have power but no authority.

NON-FINANCIAL ACTIVITIES

In order to assess Twining as an example of late-nineteenth-century philanthropy it is necessary to examine her activities, both as a member of voluntary associations and when acting alone. Her restructuring of workhouse staff aimed to give strength to, and protect, the new female workforce. When Twining unsuccessfully applied for permission to hold classes in the 1850s, she discovered the weakness of the lone reformer. Thereafter she negotiated from the stronghold of a pressure group, such as the Workhouse Visiting Society or the Workhouse Nursing Association, until her old age.

Twining used her networking skills throughout her working life. She used the family bank to place the accounts of various voluntary organisations with which she was associated. During her so-called retirement she continued to network, and took advantage of new ventures to use networks created by others for her own use. In Worthing, the committee members' names are not known to be associated in any other context with her. She started to draw the committee into a wider network: there is a donation from Mrs Henty, the treasurer's surname is Henty, and the accounts are at Henty's Bank in Worthing.[37] District nursing was a local cause and needed a local power base, not a national one. Twining supplied the drive and the experience.

The hard-working infirmary nurses trained by WNA were an important source of information for Twining. Over one hundred were employed in forty-eight workhouse infirmaries in 1897, and she entertained them in her home, as she did for her own infirmary nurses in Kensington.[38] She had opportunities to meet them at their annual meetings such as that in 1893, which sixty-five of them attended and at which she gave a speech.[39] She quoted from their letters which described their inadequate diet and their poor treatment by the master and matron.

Twining also used organisations and voluntary associations to further her work. She particularly supported the Charity Organisation Society (COS), even though she did not hold an official position in the association. She also continued to use the plethora of ground level organisations such as the Brabazon occupational therapy scheme, the Workhouse Girls Aid Committee (which helped girls after their 'first fall') and the Kyrle Society. She recorded how the antipathy of the Tunbridge Wells guardians prevented her from using the Metropolitan Association for Befriending Young Servants (MABYS) and the Girls' Friendly Society (GFS), and so she visited the workhouse girls in service herself.[40]

Her use of family and friends greatly decreased towards the end of her life. As a professional person her network now consisted of other specialists rather than people she knew by chance. However Twining did not abandon family and friends. Jane Wilson, her friend and supporter, had her credentials depicted as 'a sister having married a nephew of our dear friend Richard J. Lane'.[41] Twining continued to be an active member of the WNA even after Jane Wilson, who was a trained nurse, took over as secretary. Wilson moved to St Luke's, thus giving Twining ample opportunity to exert her influence as her public and private life merged.

Twining continued her links with Angela Burdett Coutts and, although she no longer needed her financial backing, she did use Coutts Bank for the WNA accounts. (The accounts moved back and forth from Coutts to Twinings.) Significantly, when Burdett Coutts' funeral took place in Westminster Abbey there was a simultaneous service in St Stephen's, Westminster (a church built with funds from Burdett Coutts) and the service was conducted by the Rev. W. H. G. Twining.[42]

As an elder stateswoman of philanthropy, Twining was effectively networked by associations because of her example as a working woman and as a reformer; and because of her talents and connections. Problems were therefore identified in the nursing press as 'More work for Miss Twining!' as work was publicly brought to her.[43] Hollis suggests that when the Women's Guardians Society was created, this was with Twining's 'blessings'. Although there is no mention of her having a post this does not mean that her expertise and knowledge were unused.[44] In May 1904 Twining sent the Women in Local Government Society a list of nineteen former subscribers to the Women's Guardians Society to whom the WLGS could send letters 'with her compliments'.[45] The WGS had dissolved, but this did not stop Twining utilising the archives for one of her causes. If Twining was central to organisations created and run by others, this may account for the fact that fewer names were mentioned in her later works. Her recollections of her early working life are crammed with the names of the great and the good, particularly women. If, in this later period, she was among the great and the good herself then she was being networked by others. In 1888, for example, Twining was invited (as was Octavia Hill), to be on an electoral committee dedicated to backing women standing for the London County Council and to raising money for funds, regardless of party politics.

The WGS was closely linked to other societies and organisations which reflected Twining's interests: the Workhouse Nursing Association, the Brabazon scheme, the Metropolitan Association for Befriending Young Servants, the GFS and the Boarding Out Society.[46] The WLGS approached Twining to be their president in 1904, and in a speech proposing her for a second year of tenure, Mrs Theodore Williams said that Twining was the role model which spurred her into a public life. It is clear that Twining's name as president was intended to inspire more young women.[47] She was an active president, although aware of the passing years. Her acceptance speech for re-election was reported thus: 'in a vigorous speech she caused some amusement by hazarding the doubt whether she was not inconsistent in remaining President when she had recently been protesting against the continuance in posts of old and incapable people'.[48] She resigned in 1906, aged 86, and was created vice-president.

Twining carried out her duties as Poor Law Guardian in Tunbridge Wells and Kensington conscientiously. With the exception of her last year of tenure, she attended the meetings regularly at Kensington, even when they fell on Christmas Eve. In her three years at Tunbridge Wells, she claimed to have only missed four meetings, and drew a parallel with a male guardian who only attended three meetings in a year with the comment: 'what would have been said if a woman Guardian had acted thus! Truly there is in more than one department of life, a different standard for men and women!'[49] She did her full share of the committee work and used this to pursue her other cause to further the general welfare of women, children, the elderly and the sick. As a guardian Twining attended poor law conferences (from which women guardians had initially been excluded) and these were a new opportunity for her to network in a previously exclusively male circle. She attended the annual conferences selectively, rather than automatically, and either gave a paper or spoke in response from the floor. On one occasion she was the first to reply and her response was almost as long as the paper itself.[50]

She also used journals and the press to reach interested groups such as the church reader – *Newberry House Magazine, A Threefold Cord*; the general reader – *Nineteenth Century, The National Review*; health care workers – *The Hospital*; like-minded philanthropists – *Charity Organisation Review*; and, of course, the nursing profession, the most important publication of which was *Nursing Notes*. Subtitled the 'Journal of the Workhouse Infirmary Nursing Association', *Nursing Notes* had a regular column giving not only WNA news, but also the activities of women guardians such as Louisa Twining. Twining often combined her causes such as when she wrote to *The Times* on 9 January 1904 as Vice-President of WNA and mentioned the COS. Twining was a skilled and assiduous communicator who repeatedly expressed the same ideas for a different audience, and different ideas for the same audience.

FINANCIAL ACTIVITIES

In common with other Victorians, Twining believed it was right and proper for society to support its less able members through charity. Almsgivers were not only the wealthy, and Twining held that all could give to charity regardless of class or income. Even the poorest could give something for it was not the quantity of the gift that mattered, more the act of giving. She strongly disapproved of indiscriminate almsgiving though this was partly solved by her support of the Charity Organisation Society. The COS epitomised the reaction of some philanthropists and many middle- and upper-class Victorians towards poor people who demonstrated agency in exercising their 'freedom of choice' by applying to more than one charity to meet the same need. The COS was founded to coordinate charity and to ensure that only those held to be deserving were helped, and equally that recipients received help from only one source. Louisa Twining 'thoroughly agreed' with these principles in a period during which recipients were viewed as supplicants rather than consumers. She publicly gave the COS her support and, as a poor law guardian for Kensington, was automatically an *ex-officio* member of the local committee. The committee met regularly at the workhouse and was used by the guardians to coordinate outdoor relief.[51]

Twining also had opinions on pay for women's work. Her earliest schemes for nursing were influenced by the deaconess movement. She noted in 1861 that pay for nurses was not believed necessary on the continent but that she thought 'the present means of subsistence and a prospect of future maintenance in old age' would be 'sufficient inducement' in Britain.[52] Eventually, she believed in payment even during training, saying it was 'absolutely necessary' to pay probationers salaries of not less than £10 a year.[53]

She perceived rightly that her client groups were fluid and, realising that nurses become old, she wanted them paid enough to save for old age, but not so much that individuals could be attracted to the work by the pay alone. Finally, she floated the idea of a pension, which was available to some military nurses, with the caveat of a contract of several years to amortise costs.[54] In Kensington when she was a guardian, a nurse retired 'due to Disease of the Knee, the loss of one eye and repeated indisposition', and was given a pension.[55]

Twining used her own wealth for the benefit of others. She inherited £17,000 on the death of her parents in 1857 and 1866, and this gave her the freedom to pursue her philanthropic ideals without alienating her social circle. Her banking background is evident in the importance she attached to the accuracy of the financial accounts of charitable societies. Twining consistently donated money to the organisations for which she worked: she gave £100 to WNA for a special appeal, but usually it was less than £10 for causes such as the welfare of the feeble-minded, or promoting women in local elections.[56] She believed that money, whatever its source, should be used with care. When she travelled in her capacity as a Poor Law Guardian for Kensington to inspect outlying schools or convalescent homes in Margate she never travelled first class, unlike her male colleagues. She was conscious that the rates were other people's money which had been hard-earned and that she therefore had a duty to spend it wisely.[57]

Her personal belief was that donations or alms should be freely given without any exchange taking place. This meant a rejection of bazaars and entertainments, common ways of raising funds at this time. Having rejected the common fund-raising methods, what did she do? The voluntary societies with which she was associated published the customary lists of donations and subscription by name and amount. These served two purposes: the accounts were easily accessible for inspection, and peer group pressure was likely to entice more people to subscribe and to enhance the amount they gave. When, in 1880, Twining gave £10 to the WNA, Florence Nightingale also made a donation, of 10 guineas.[58]

In this period Twining deliberately reduced her work with parish-based associations such as Temperance Societies and Mother's Meetings, and so was no longer able to draw personally on their individual members for funds. Previously she had sent copies of societies' annual reports to targeted individuals to gain financial and other forms of support. There are copies of WNA reports in Florence Nightingale's personal papers, complete with red pencil marks. Thus far there is less evidence of mail shots in the late nineteenth century than for the earlier part of Twining's working life.

The income of voluntary societies came from regular subscriptions (usually annual) and donations. Individuals often gave in both categories. The income was a mixture of public and private donations, but predominantly private. By 1891 the WNA received subscriptions from twenty-four Boards of Guardians, and in 1891 the Worthing District Nursing Association received a payment of £10 from the East Preston Guardians, almost an eighth of its income.[59]

The WNA, founded in 1879, trained over one hundred probationers and had appointed nearly 300 staff by 1890.[60] Created to improve nursing in workhouse infirmaries, it eventually appreciated that it could not supply sufficient numbers to meet the demand by the unions. Not only was the work arduous and suitable candidates hard to find, but the large amount of capital needed was not forthcoming from subscriptions and donations. In a series of tense meetings at the end of 1897, the association debated its future as it realised the 'impossibility of adequately meeting, by private effort alone, the demand for trained nurses'.[61] In a further meeting Twining proposed the second resolution, that the association should not dissolve, and that it was 'The State Department's duty to provide nurses for workhouse infirmaries'. She hoped that if the WNA stopped their piecemeal effort to provide trained infirmary nurses then the local government board would feel obliged to do so on a much larger scale.[62]

Here, in a shift in her philosophy, Twining unambiguously argued that the state should be responsible for providing not only the workhouse infirmary, but also its professional staff. Moreover, it had a duty to do so. Philanthropy created the trained infirmary nurse, and it now desired that the state should accept responsibility for their training because the financial demands could not be met by private money topped up by local Boards of Guardians. The WNA had created a demand which it could not possibly hope to meet. Twining's reaction not only set a limitation on welfare provision by charity, but also demonstrated her belief that the voluntary sector could work in harmony with the state.

CONCLUSION

Louisa Twining was an accomplished operator of the women's philanthropic network. This brought together women with common and overlapping causes, whose public and private lives also overlapped. Social events became opportunities for furthering philanthropic work not only among themselves, but also among the men in their social circle. Just as men used the old-boy network of family, school, university and gentlemen's clubs, so women like Twining used the old-girls' network of family, philanthropic work and voluntary organisations. Family, friends, and co-workers could be one and the same and were found within all parts of the network.

Twining's life has been defined as 'a life devoted to the service of society'.[63] The use of the word 'service' is significant, because of its implications of welfare and benevolence. Twining remained concerned with the welfare of women, children, the elderly and the sick under the care of the poor law. During a period of so-called retirement, she chiefly championed her other, related cause, of the professionalisation of women's work. Here she could achieve the welfare she desired for her chosen groups, through women providers and managers.

Her personal approach to work did not change. Twining told her followers that they should persevere, be prompt, and be punctual, as indeed she was.[64] The *Nursing Record* described her as a 'veteran pioneer of workhouse reform' and as 'indefatigable'.[65] She was concerned with long-term gains and realised the importance of the work being respected by men. She was also aware of the reputation of some ladies' committees and protested their worth and good work. Twining still gave without expecting a return, always for welfare or women's work. In her will she left legacies to a broad range of charities such as Home Missions for the Church of England, nurse training for the sick poor, and Nursing Sisters of St John the Divine.

Many of her ideas were those of her youth and middle years, but some did change, for example those on nurses' pay and the role of the state in the provision of welfare and in nurse training. She appreciated that her client groups were not fixed, that nurses could become sick unless employed fairly and that they, in time, would become old. She lessened her emphasis on religion in public and talked less of women's duty to care for the sick, and more of their inherent skill, even if the language of their 'sacred calling' was still that of religion. Her religion became more private but no less important as a personal force. She did, however, not now expect it of others.

Twining had a shrewd understanding of how organisations of all sizes worked, although her personal experience was limited to working in either small organisations or voluntary associations in which there were flattened hierarchies that allowed the strongest personalities to emerge as leaders. She also saw the necessity for poor law nurses to have their own management tree based on a vertical hierarchy, not only to protect them from the interference from non-health care personnel, but also to make them more effective by giving them authority. The Boards of Guardians were power-based, with a chairman and the remainder equal in status, though in practice some were always more equal than others. She also understood the relationship between occupations (such as those between workhouse and nursing staff), between appointed staff and consultants (workhouse staff and the doctor or chaplain) and between official workers and unofficial workers (workhouse staff and lady visitors).

Twining was, above all, pragmatic about what she believed could be achieved. She wrote that 'Many are even now grasping at distant objects beyond their reach, while duties, numerous and important, waiting to be performed are within the power of everyone.'[66] Her personal work style was cautious. In Tunbridge Wells she records that she wrote in the report book for seven months that 'everything was satisfactory and in good order (which I was tempted to suggest might be stereotyped to save trouble)'. She then entered two pages of suggestions, waited for the 'storm and opposition', but instead a sub-committee was formed consisting of herself and two friendly guardians, and all was duly sorted out to her satisfaction.[67] But caution should not be mistaken for timidity. She was described by her contemporary, that larger-than-life character Frances Power Cobbe, as 'General Twining'.[68]

But now she shared the publicity with other women, many much younger than herself, and she was aware of the gap between herself and the next generation of workers. She wrote that her successors 'deliberately ignored' her experience and that of her fellow workers, with the result that much precious time was lost. She was 'quite sure that this spirit did not prevail to the same extent formerly'.[69] Unlike the pre-1882 period of her life, it is noticeable how she repeatedly withdrew from work: she resigned from posts such as secretary of the WNA and president of the WLGS, and moved house several times thus preventing her from standing for re-election as a guardian. This may, of course, have less to do with tensions with her new co-workers, and more to do with her age and her awareness of her own mortality. 'She hinted at this' in a letter to *The Times* in 1907 which referred to 'this, perhaps my last communication'.[70] She lived a further five years during which time she continued to write letters on women in local government, poor law reform, and the care of the feeble-minded.

This later period of her working life is very different though, because of her official posts as a Poor Law Guardian and as a role model and leader of elected women. Twining's posts as poor law guardian represent an important change in her working life. Previously, she had worked solely in the voluntary sector, but as a local government official she crossed a personal Rubicon and took an established position. These posts as guardian were also significant in that they challenged the men who thought this space was solely theirs. The status of these established positions placed her equal to her professionally qualified brothers, through her own merits rather than by consanguinity. Her search for self-esteem and self-actualisation, both motivating forces as much as her Christianity, drove her to overcome her gendered childhood.

This is a period which has been identified as that of the professionalising of philanthropy.[71] Whether Twining's emphasis on national standards, state recognition and a carefully selected and trained workforce presaged a professional society is the subject of further research.[72] The late nineteenth century saw the fruition of many of the proposals set out in her *Workhouses and Women's Work* in 1857. In this she described her earliest ideas for a professional body of women.[73] She waited half a century for some of them; she was patient, specific and cautious and chose her moments. And her patience was rewarded. In 1912 she wrote to *The Times* welcoming the poor law changes which she had sought in 1863. She reminded the readers that she had been a poor law guardian, the originator of the WVS and WNA, and that at the beginning of her working life when she was 'the only visitor to the poor lonely inmates, . . . [and that] . . . the helplessness and misery of their then condition can hardly be imagined now'.[74] Eight days later, aged almost 92, she died.

NOTES

1 I wish to thank Mr S. H. G. Twining, of R. Twining & Co. Ltd, for the loan of pamphlets written by Louisa Twining. Thanks are also due to Miss Wilma MacPherson, Director of Nursing of the Guy's and St Thomas's Hospital Trust, for permission to refer to the Florence Nightingale Collection in the Greater London Record Office. I am also grateful to Pat Thane and Jessica Cooke for their comments on this chapter.

2 See, for example, Brian Abel-Smith, *A History of the Nursing Profession*, London, Heinemann, 1960; M. A. Crowther, *The Workhouse System 1834–1929*, London, Methuen, 1983; Patricia Hollis, *Ladies Elect*, Oxford, Oxford University Press, 1989; Julia Parker, *Women and Welfare: Ten Victorian Women in Public Social Service*, Basingstoke, Macmillan, 1989; Prochaska, *Women and Philanthropy*; Martha Vicinus, *Independent Women: Work and Community for Single Women 1850–1920*, London, Virago, 1985.

3 Kathleen E. McCrone, 'Feminism and Philanthropy in Victorian England: the Case of Louisa Twining', *Canadian Historical Association: Historical Papers*, 1976, pp. 123–39. Twining is also one of the ten women in Parker, *Women and Welfare*.

4 Frank Prochaska, 'Philanthropy', in F. M. L. Thompson (ed.), *The Cambridge Social History of Britain 1750–1950*, vol. 3, Cambridge, Cambridge University Press, 1993, pp. 359, 384.

5 This has been noted in Anne Summers, 'A Home from Home: Women's Philanthropic Work in the Nineteenth Century', in S. Burman (ed.), *Fit Work for Women*, London, Croom Helm, 1979, p. 36.

6 She knew no families with governesses although she did know some who sent their girls to boarding school. Louisa Twining, *Recollections of Life and Work*, London, Edward Arnold, 1893, pp. 17–23.

7 Ibid., pp. 20 and 152–3.

8 Ibid.
9 Twining acknowledges the educational influences of her brothers Aldred and William during her early years because of the way they guided her reading. She carefully omits to mention Richard: ibid., pp. 27–8.
10 For Elizabeth Twining and the Mother's Meeting movement in general see: Frank Prochaska, 'A Mother's Country: Mother's Meetings and Family Welfare in Britain 1850–1950', *History*, 1989, vol. 74, pp. 379–99.
11 Twining, *Recollections*, p. 111.
12 For the importance of these factors in a biographical study see: Carolyn Steedman, *Childhood, Culture, and Class in Britain: Margaret McMillan, 1860–1931*, London, Virago Press, 1990.
13 The Society was part of the Social Science Association. For the importance of the Association, particularly to female reformers, see Kathleen E. McCrone, 'The National Association for the Promotion of Social Science and the Advancement of Victorian Women', *Atlantis*, 1982, vol. 8, pp. 44–66.
14 Twining's suggestion that women were suitable to be poor law guardians has been noted in Frank Prochaska, *Women and Philanthropy in Nineteenth Century England*, Oxford, Oxford University Press, 1980, p. 80.
15 She was involved with many other associations such as the Association for Promoting Cottage Training Homes for Workhouse Children, the National Association for the Care of the Feeble Minded and the Metropolitan and National Association which was concerned with district nursing.
16 Frank Prochaska, *The Voluntary Impulse: Philanthropy in Modern Britain*, London, Faber & Faber, p. 7; this is further developed in Prochaska, *Philanthropy*.
17 Pat Thane, 'Later Victorian Women', in T. R. Gourvish and Alan O'Day (eds), *Later Victorian Britain 1867–1900*, Basingstoke, Macmillan, 1990, p. 190.
18 Minutes of the Strand Board of Guardians, 10 May 1853.
19 Twining, *Recollections*, p. 257.
20 Twining quotes this definition without naming the source in: L. Twining, *Charity at the End of the Nineteenth Century*, London, Westminster Church Press, 1901, reprinted from *The Charity Organisation Reporter*, 1884, p. 1.
21 Ibid., p. 2.
22 Louisa Twining, 'Women as Public Servants', *Nineteenth Century*, 1890, vol. 28, p. 952.
23 Louisa Twining, 'Fifty Years of Women's Work', *The National Review*, 1887, vol. IX, p. 661. This was later published as a pamphlet and retitled 'Women's Work Official and Unofficial', publisher and date unknown.
24 Louisa Twining, 'Women as Public Servants', *Nineteenth Century*, 1890, vol. 28, p. 952.
25 Louisa Twining, *Nursing in Workhouses: A Paper Read before the*

Ladies Conference, Liverpool, 1891, Liverpool, Gilbert G. Walmsley, 1892, p. 8.
26 Twining, 'Fifty Years', p. 660.
27 Anna Jameson, *The Communion of Labour: A Second Lecture on the Social Employments of Women*, London, Longman, Brown, Green, Longman & Roberts, 1856.
28 Twining, 'Women as Public Servants', p. 952.
29 Louisa Twining, *Workhouses and Pauperism and Women's Work in the Administration of the Poor Law*, London, Methuen, 1898, p. x.
30 For example see Twining, *Recollections*, p. 281.
31 Twining, *Workhouses*, p. 130, and *Recollections*, p. 258.
32 Twining, 'Women as Public Servants', p. 953.
33 Twining, *Workhouses*, p. 182, and 'Fifty Years', p. 663.
34 Twining, 'Fifty Years', p. 663.
35 Louisa Twining quoted in *Nursing Record*, 20 December 1902.
36 Twining, *Workhouses*, p. 122.
37 *First Report of the Worthing District Nursing Association*, 1892.
38 See Twining's evidence to the Select Committee of the House of Lords on Metropolitan Hospitals, 1891, 22642–798; also Twining, *Workhouses*, pp. 189–211; *The Times*, 3 December 1897; Twining, *Recollections*, p. 261.
39 *Nursing Notes*, 1 July 1893.
40 Twining, *Workhouses*, p. 134.
41 Twining, *Recollections*, p. 240.
42 *The Times*, 7 January 1907.
43 *The Nursing Record*, 13 June 1889. Jurors at a Belfast coroners court recommended that there should be more paid nurses at the infirmary following the death of John M'Sorley in the Belfast Union due to delirium tremens.
44 Hollis, *Ladies*, p. 231.
45 WLGS Minutes, 17 May 1904.
46 This point has been made by Hollis, *Ladies*, p. 234.
47 Twining was the third choice for President. Lady Battersea and Mrs Arthur Lyttelton both declined the position: Minutes of the WLGS, 16 February 1905 and 22 March 1904.
48 *Report of Annual General Meeting of the WLGS*, 16 March 1905.
49 Twining, *Workhouses*, p. 153; quoted in Hollis, *Ladies*, p. 214.
50 Central Poor Law Conference 1896, pp. 68–71.
51 *15th Annual Report of the COS*, 1884; *17th Annual Report of the COS*, 1886.
52 Louisa Twining, *Nurses for the Sick with a Letter to Young Women*, London, Longman, Green, Longman & Roberts, 1861, p. 17.
53 Second Annual Report of the WNA, 1881.
54 Twining, *Workhouses*, p. 215.
55 *Minutes of the Kensington Board of Guardians*, 10 December 1885.
56 *12th Report of the Workhouse Nursing Association*, 1891; *Accounts of the National Association for Promoting the Welfare of the Feeble Minded*, 1889; obituary of Louisa Twining, 12th Annual General Meeting of WLGS, 1913.

57 Obituary of Louisa Twining in *Nursing Notes*, November 1912; Twining, *Workhouses*, p. 116.
58 *WNA, Second Annual Report*, 1881. As the WNA records are incomplete, it is not possible to draw wider conclusions.
59 WNA, 1891; *First Report of the Worthing District Nursing Association*, 1892.
60 WNA, 1891, quoted in Hollis, *Ladies*, p. 272.
61 *The Nursing Record*, 6 November 1897.
62 Twining's resolution that the WNA should continue as a centre of information for guardians and nurses as well as for its own nurses was passed: *Nursing Notes*, 1 February 1898.
63 David Owen, *English Philanthropy 1660–1960*, London, Oxford University Press, 1965, pp. 1, 394. Owen's examination of philanthropy only includes individuals who made substantial pecuniary benefactions and Louisa Twining is cited as an example of the 'lives of service to society' which were excluded from his study. As few women had control over very large amounts of money this definition dismisses nearly all women's philanthropic work as well as most of that of middle- and working-class men.
64 Louisa Twining, *Recollections of Workhouse Visiting and Management*, London, Kegan Paul, 1880, pp. xi–xii.
65 *Nursing Record*, 8 March 1902 and 14 June 1888.
66 Twining, 'Fifty Years', p. 660.
67 Twining, *Workhouses*, p. 136.
68 Frances Power Cobbe, *Life of Frances Power Cobbe as Told by Herself*, London, Swan Sonnenschein, 1904, p. 319.
69 Twining, *Workhouses*, p. ix.
70 *The Times*, 11 January 1907.
71 Hollis, *Ladies*, p. 201.
72 These issues will be discussed in my forthcoming thesis.
73 Twining, *Recollections of Workhouse Visiting*, Appendix VI, pp. 138–96.
74 *The Times*, 17 September 1912.

Chapter 6

The campaign for birth control in Britain in the 1920s

Lesley Hoggart

In 1922 Nurse Daniels was dismissed by Edmonton District Council for the offence of distributing birth control information. The Ministry of Health responded to angry demands for her reinstatement with the following ruling:

> The Maternity and Child Welfare Centres should deal only with the expectant or nursing mother and infant and not with the married or unmarried woman contemplating the application of contraceptive methods.

> It is not the function of an ante-natal centre to give advice in regard to birth control, and exceptional cases where the avoidance of pregnancy seems desirable on medical grounds should be referred for particular advice to a private practitioner or hospital.[1]

This unequivocal ruling against the provision of birth control information precipitated a campaign which aimed specifically at persuading the Ministry to reverse their position.[2]

The birth control campaign was fought on many fronts. In the House of Commons, supporters of birth control bombarded successive Ministers of Health with questions, deputations and petitions requesting that the ruling be reversed. The Ministers' responses rarely varied: they declared that such a decision could only be made with parliamentary approval because a significant proportion of the population disapproved of birth control. In 1926, the Labour MP Ernest Thurtle's Ten Minute Bill in favour of birth control failed to gain Commons approval while, in the same year, a similar motion in the House of Lords was successful.

Events in Parliament were more than matched by constant activity throughout Britain. Local authorities were targeted with letters, petitions and deputations asking them to take initiatives which might aid the birth control campaign. Campaigners, such as Marie Stopes, Stella Browne and Dora Russell, were engaged on countless speaking tours. Voluntary birth control clinics were established. Large public meetings and conferences were held. One clear indication of the scale of interest in birth control in this period was the estimate in 1929 that since the First World War fifteen million books, pamphlets and brochures on contraception had become available in England.[3]

It is generally accepted that the campaign succeeded when there was an abrupt policy reversal in 1930.[4] The Ministry of Health, semi-secretly and without parliamentary approval, issued Memorandum 153/MCW which authorised local authorities to permit birth control advice '[i]n cases where further pregnancy would be detrimental to health'.[5] The birth control campaign that preceded this policy reversal brought together a number of different organisations with distinct, and often contradictory, political attitudes. It is here argued that birth control was both a class and a gender issue in the 1920s. A variety of feminist ideas were evident in that, for example, many of the women activists were committed to sexual liberation. It was not, however, simply a feminist campaign. Class considerations were of paramount importance. Voluntary clinics openly targeted working-class women and, for the first time, working-class women's organisations campaigned for birth control as a right already enjoyed by the middle class. While much has been written about the politics and activity of the Malthusian League and Marie Stopes, very little work has been published on the involvement of working-class women.[6] In what follows emphasis will be laid on an organisation which did encompass working-class involvement, the Workers' Birth Control Group (WBCG), an organisation formed specifically to campaign on birth control in the Labour movement. The WBCG attempted to combine feminism and socialism and successfully mobilised working-class women and men.[7]

The chapter has three main purposes: first, to show how the politics of the WBCG overcame working-class hostility towards birth control; second, to show that birth control was both a feminist and a socialist issue while revealing contradictions between these two political approaches; third, to assess the difficulties the WBCG faced in campaigning within the Labour Party. This final section discusses and challenges the commonly held assumption that gender divisions provide an adequate explanation for the persistent opposition of the Labour Party leadership.[8] It examines national and local campaign activity, and contends that the Labour Party's pursuit of electoral success was also a significant factor. (See also Chapter 7.)

THE WORKERS' BIRTH CONTROL GROUP

At the 1924 Annual Conference of Labour Women a special 'unofficial' conference on birth control was held. Two hundred delegates attended and formed the Workers' Birth Control Group. Membership was open to men and women members of the Labour Party and affiliated bodies and members of the Co-operative Guild.[9] The women who had organised this initiative believed that a new body was necessary to concentrate on campaigning for positive government policy on birth control.

> The Group did not wish to work in antagonism to existing birth control organisations but distinguished itself from them in its political aim, its emphasis on propaganda to obtain public action, rather than on the attempt to establish separate clinics and give information in that manner and through pamphlets.[10]

Their basic political analysis was also quite different from those who had pioneered the development of voluntary birth control clinics: Marie Stopes and the Malthusian League.

In 1921 Stopes had formed the Society for Constructive Birth Control and Racial Progress and, shortly after, opened Britain's first birth control clinic. Her political approach combined a radical attitude towards sexuality, conservative eugenics and blatant class prejudice.[11] The Malthusian League, formed in 1877, opened the second birth control clinic in November 1921. The League accepted Malthus' basic premise that poverty was caused by overpopulation but, unlike Malthus, advocated birth control as a population control measure. They maintained a hostility towards working-class aspirations for social reforms which was mirrored by working-class hostility towards any proposals that might be touched by the ghost of Malthus.[12]

The WBCG therefore set out to emphasise that their politics were quite different:

> We now formed our Workers' Birth Control Group to make clear that we were working in and with the Labour Party and

did not share the views of the extreme Malthusians, or the Eugenists' notion that the poor were inferior stock.[13]

The WBCG found that it was not easy to overcome socialist distrust of Malthusian doctrines. The Labour movement was slow to become involved in the birth control campaign in the 1920s. When the first voluntary clinics opened in 1921 they were not mentioned in *Labour Woman*, nor was the issue discussed at the women's conference that year. This is despite the fact that these clinics were aimed at working-class women. In 1922, the year in which the Ministry of Health issued the circular which prompted the campaign, *Labour Woman* was completely silent. At their conference in 1922, the women discussed in some detail reforms they thought the state should initiate to meet the needs of women and children, but these did not include birth control.

There was a level of genuine confusion among many Labour women who were not necessarily opposed to birth control but were ambivalent about whether it was necessary. In particular, the belief that socialism and birth control were in some ways contradictory lingered. A good example of the dilemma facing many politically active working-class women was expressed by Lillie Turner in a letter to *Labour Woman* in 1924:

> We, as Labour and Socialist Women, are out first of all for a new social order, and we believe that through our practical Socialist programme we can achieve a full and free life for every man, woman, and child . . .

> I fully and entirely agree that the question of birth control should not be dragged into the public arena. Let us put first things first, and get on with our particular job of establishing the Socialist Commonwealth.[14]

Anti-Malthusian arguments were often used as an excuse by those who, for quite different reasons, were opposed to adopting a positive attitude towards birth control as Labour policy. The party leadership was afraid of embracing such a controversial policy and one of their tactics for evading the issue was to declare that birth control was no solution to the problems faced by working-class women. The WBCG recognised that these objections had some resonance, and therefore took pains to stress that they did not propose birth control as an answer to social problems but as part of a social reform programme. They made a conscious, and largely successful, effort to distance themselves from neo-Malthusianism. There is evidence that the attitude of many Labour Party members changed during the decade, possibly due to the activity of the WBCG. At the Labour Party Conference in 1926 Ramsay MacDonald raised the spectre of population control, asking: 'Are you to commit the Labour Party to neo-Malthusianism?' The speech was, in the words of Marion Phillips (Woman Organiser of the Labour Party and editor of *Labour Woman*), 'Curiously ineffective'.[15] The formation of the WBCG, which posed birth control as a socialist issue, was a major breakthrough for the campaign.

The Workers' Birth Control Group and socialism

World War I was followed by a period of intense class struggle which continued until 1926.[16] This was accompanied by a revival of fortunes for socialists. The Labour Party was one beneficiary of the changing political climate, being accepted as the official opposition in 1922 and in January 1924 forming its first ever government. The Independent Labour Party (ILP) also benefited, reaching the height of its influence in the period 1922 to 1925.[17] One consequence of the class polarisation was the movement of many women, most of whom tried to maintain a commitment to feminist ideals, into the Labour movement.[18] Many members of the WBCG were committed socialists, a considerable number being members of the ILP which adopted a positive attitude towards women's issues.[19]

The WBCG connected the struggle for birth control with social-ist aims. In direct contrast to the Malthusian League and Marie Stopes, the WBCG argued that social reforms were necessary to alleviate the poverty and appalling living conditions of the working class. They concentrated on reforms which they believed could improve the lives of working-class mothers,[20] and often provided detailed recommendations in their political interventions. A policy document submitted by the WBCG in 1925 to the Royal Commission on National Health Insurance did not just propose birth control, but dealt also with the question of maternal health within the context of the general social conditions facing working-class women. The memorandum discussed the persistence of a high maternal death rate and ill-health associated with pregnancy, specifically mortality from puerperal sepsis connected with abortion. It made recommendations on housing needs; commented on the lack of maternity beds; and called for improvements in the medical service and employment conditions stressing their influence on maternal morbidity.[21] Overall birth control was, for the WBCG, part of a programme of social reform, not an alternative. It was, however, an essential part: the WBCG believed that social progress depended upon women enjoying the freedom to control their fertility. This was made clear in one of their stated objectives:

> To strengthen public opinion among workers as to the importance of Birth Control in any scheme of social progress.[22]

The WBCG put a great deal of effort into arguing that the Labour Party, as a socialist organisation, should support the campaign for birth control, specifically pressing the claims of the working mother. One particular approach adopted by the WBCG was to argue that they sought to improve the conditions of work of the working-class mother in much the same way as trade unions sought to improve the conditions of work of their members. At the 1926 Labour Party Conference these arguments carried extra weight in the light of the women's support of the miners during the lockout. Dora Russell very deliberately drew parallels:

> She wanted them to realise that to the women it was as important as the seven-hour day was to the Miners, and their opinion ought to have the same weight as the Miners' Federation had in their matters.[23]

In the same year Ernest Thurtle MP, a supporter of the WBCG, pleaded for his Ten Minute Bill as a socialist measure to help working-class women. At the 1927 Labour Party Conference Mrs Lawther, herself a miner's wife, declared that she had worked fifteen years in industry and always been an active trade unionist. She then turned towards the miners and asked:

> Surely you will not turn the women down on this question, because it was the women who stood four square with you in your dispute. It is four times as dangerous to bear a child as it is for you to go down a mine. You are seeking legislation to make your occupation safe; will you still go on allowing your wives to suffer under this ban?[24]

The WBCG also thought that socialists should campaign for the state to provide birth control information. Working-class women were being discriminated against by the very nature of the health service then available. Although it was also not easy for middle-class women to receive birth control advice, working-class women were at a disadvantage in that they were entirely dependent upon the public health service, where giving advice was forbidden. Members of the WBCG therefore argued that class discrimination was taking place. Dorothy Jewson, for example, asked the Labour Minister of Health, John Wheatley, in the Commons in July 1924, whether he was aware that

> [m]any working-class women attending these welfare centres are unfit to bear children and to bring up healthy children and the doctors know they are unfit, and yet they are unable to give this information, which any upper- or middle-class woman can obtain from a private doctor?[25]

The Ministry of Health's position was that women whose health was so poor that they should avoid another pregnancy could go to a private doctor or hospital. The WBCG countered this by saying that because birth control was a matter of public health, women should not have to rely upon private doctors; that hospitals were not state institutions; and that working-class women could not afford to pay for the information they so badly needed.[26] Their publicity material demanded the provision of free birth control information within the public health service. The request for equal access was also one of the most frequent appeals made by speakers at the Conferences of Labour Women. In 1924 Mrs Jones from Greenwich made this point forcefully.

> The wealthy woman says how many children she can have because she can afford to pay for the knowledge, and we say that the working mother should be able to get the knowledge although she has no money.[27]

The Workers' Birth Control Group and feminism

After women were granted a limited parliamentary suffrage in 1918, feminists did not simply rest on their laurels. In the 1920s, many became involved in a number of different campaigns on issues that affected women directly and an alliance of feminism and social welfare emerged which dominated the inter-war years.[28] One important aspect of this 'new feminism' was the involvement of working-class women's organisations in these social welfare campaigns, most of which sought to improve maternal and infant welfare.[29] (See also Chapter 3.)

Successive governments were also concerned with maternal and infant welfare and initiated reforms which were directed towards working-class families. The reforms were accompanied by a prescriptive ideology of motherhood, which emphasised the importance of healthy and intelligent motherhood to an imperial nation, and were designed in the interests of infant, rather than maternal, welfare.[30] By contrast, the 'new feminism' concentrated upon the needs of mothers. The WBCG shared this approach. They focused on the needs of working-class mothers and incorporated birth control demands into their own framework for infant and maternal welfare.

Many feminists who were to campaign around birth control in the 1970s proposed sexual liberation and argued for the need to challenge the sexual division of labour. They often expressed disappointment with the result of the birth control campaign of the 1920s. Sheila Rowbotham, for instance, has argued that the outcome of the campaign did not reflect the politics of the socialist-feminists involved: women did not gain control over their biological destiny but merely succeeded in establishing the new ideology of 'family planning'.[31] This analysis involves an over-estimation of the extent to which the birth control campaigners sought to overturn women's biological destiny. The most radical ideas did not guide the campaign and the activists, even when challenging contemporary prejudices, remained fundamentally bound to their own era. This will be particularly clear when considering their attitudes towards motherhood and sexuality.

The Organisation of Labour Women stressed the needs of working-class mothers. They promoted a feminism which valued marriage and motherhood and they strove to raise the status of this occupation.[32] The WBCG largely shared this outlook and incorporated it into their political approach. The membership of the WBCG was open to men and women from labour organisations '[b]ut, so far as possible, control of its policy was to be in the hands of men and women who had known the responsibility of parenthood. ... It is those who love children and care most satisfactorily for their own, who are the strongest and most eloquent advocates of birth control.'[33] The first circular which gave details of the proposed meeting at the Conference of Labour

Women listed Rose Witcop-Aldred, Marjory Allen, Frida Laski, Joan Malleson, L. L'Estrange Malone and Dora Russell as members of the provisional committee, and made a point of stating that 'All of them have children of their own'.[34] When the WBCG was formed, the only single woman on the committee was Dorothy Jewson MP and that was because there were no married Labour women in the House of Commons.[35]

The WBCG accepted women's maternal role:

> The attitude of the Group throughout is to demand knowledge, science and research for women into all problems affecting them as mothers, and recognition of their work and its importance to the community. Its members felt that their attitude on birth control, and on sex information goes hand in hand with the programme of Labour women for improved maternity care and pensions for mothers. The battle will not be fought to a successful conclusion without some degree of pugnacious feminism on the part of mothers, who were somewhat neglected in the feminist fight in the last fifty years.[36]

Even Stella Browne, possibly the most radical of the birth control campaigners, did not challenge this retention of a belief in the sexual division of labour.[37] Early in the campaign she expressed the belief, in a communication to Dora Russell, that clinics should combine maternal and infant care with contraceptive work.[38]

By far the most common argument used with reference to the needs of women within the sphere of motherhood concerned maternal health.

> Many doctors to-day, consulted privately, will admit that it is nothing short of vile cruelty to refuse the knowledge of contraceptives to women whose mental and physical health, and, in many cases, environment and economic circumstances, make it impossible for them to produce healthy children, still less to lead tolerable lives themselves.[39]

The campaign for birth control, however, by its very nature raised issues concerning sexuality. This made it a radical campaign for the 1920s. As Linda Gordon has noted, a morality which separates sex from reproduction is necessary for the acceptance of birth control.[40] The campaign for birth control in the 1920s marked a step in this direction:

> We were trying to set sex free from the stigma of sin, we saw
> it as an expression of the union and harmony of two lovers;
> our adversaries' dogma demanded that sex be indulged in only
> for the procreation of children.[41]

The 1920s witnessed greater sexual freedom and a correspon-
ding debate about sexuality and sexual morality.[42] This was,
however, tempered by persistent worries, especially by politicians
and the Church, about declining morals and the breakup of
family life.[43] One of the main opponents of improved birth control
knowledge, Dr Mary Scharlieb, expressed a common fear:

> Limitation of families is wrong and dangerous because it does
> not control nor discipline sexual passion, but by removing the
> fear of consequences it does away with the chief controlling
> and steadying influence of sexual life.[44]

In addition, the campaign specifically raised the question of
women controlling their own fertility. In some of their publicity
material and in letters to local health authorities the WBCG urged
that birth control information be available to 'those who seek it',
thus specifically calling for birth control on request.[45] Such
demands raised a great deal of opposition, which alerted the
WBCG to the controversial nature of their proposals.

The birth control campaigners in the Labour Party worked
within a framework in which there was a perceived need to stress
their lack of radicalism. In 1923, a full page in *Labour Woman*
was given over to a letter from Ethel Carroll in which she made
clear what she believed were the main concerns for Labour
women. The letter was designed to refute the charges that Labour
and socialism were out to destroy 'home life'. She raised the issue
of birth control:

> [a]ny Labour Woman who advocates birth control does so, not
> to help free love, but to help overburdened parents to limit
> their offspring according to their means, thereby helping them
> to bring up their families properly nourished and decently
> housed and clothed.[46]

Some of the women involved in the birth control campaign held
very radical views on sexuality. Individuals such as Stella Browne
and Dora Russell, who were also active in the World League for
Sexual Reform, did not, however, press all their views in the birth

control campaign. This is almost certainly because they felt they had to try to remain respectable.[47] The promotion of freer sexuality was not easily visible in the material produced by the WBCG. On the contrary, some handwritten notes by Dora Russell for the WBCG's *Memorandum to the Ministry of Health* in 1924 bear significant differences to the final, presented form. In the section on birth control and morality she expressed her own view that 'young people of eighteen should be told the facts of life by responsible people'.[48] This is not included in the same section in the final memorandum:

> Without proceeding to argue as to the definition of immorality, or the extent to which sex information should be given to young people, may we point out that the request made in this petition is the surest safeguard of morality that could have been devised. Women who seek advice at Welfare and Ante-Natal Centres are married women already pregnant or with one or more children.[49]

In their publicity material, the WBCG confined their proposals in favour of a less restricted sexuality to the marriage relationship:

> The sex love of man and woman is not only a beautiful thing in itself, strengthening the other manifestations of love that have their part in the marriage relation, but it is a health-giving thing also.[50]

Both the socialism and the feminism of the WBCG influenced their key strategy which was to try to commit a future Labour government to improve working-class women's access to birth control. They believed that the achievement of their aims depended upon convincing the entire Labour Party of the justice of their cause and the importance of the reform for working-class women. The WBCG was therefore concerned to play down arguments about sexual liberation and emphasise maternal welfare. They did not set out to destroy 'home life' and certainly took pains to keep the ideals of 'motherhood' at the forefront of the campaign. The WBCG's campaign for birth control was located firmly within the welfare feminism of the 1920s.

The WBCG rapidly discovered that such a 'moderate' framework did not succeed in quelling opposition. They were forced to realise that the Labour Party was unable to include a commitment to such a potentially contentious reform within their vision of socialism. The WBCG had hoped that Labour would support this demand of working-class women and were disappointed when the policy decided at the women's conference was rejected at the main Party Conference:

> The Labour Women supposed, until this controversy broke their confidence, that their Conference would carry the same weight in the Councils of the movement on women's questions as the miners on a mining question. It did not occur to us that a party claiming to stand for sex equality, and for scientific organisation of workers according to their job, would take up so short-sighted and unenlightened attitude on the job of a mother.[51]

Their disappointment at the lack of support was probably most acute because they believed they were arguing for a reform that was reasonable, indeed moderate. The WBCG expended most of their energy on this campaign in the Labour Party. The following section will examine the difficulties they faced.

The campaign in the Labour Party

The WBCG's attempts to enlist the support of the Labour Party were constantly frustrated. Socialist antagonism towards Malthusian doctrines was gradually overcome as working-class women demanded birth control information for themselves. There were, however, two further factors creating resistance. First, the fact that men dominated the decision-making mechanisms in the Labour Party meant that the WBCG had an uphill task in their endeavour to commit the Party to a measure which seemed to be of concern only to women. Second, the controversial nature of an issue which not only threatened established conventions regarding female sexuality, but brought private sexuality into the public arena, made it unpopular with a Party intent on making an electoral breakthrough.

Male dominance

The WBCG was well aware that part of the reason for their lack of success was the relative lack of strength of women in the Labour Party.[52] When the women lost the vote on birth control at the 1925 Conference, Dorothy Jewson was dismayed that an issue that was important for mothers had been deemed unimportant by fathers within the Labour Party:

> Even at the Conference, if there had been a good as representation of mothers as there was of fathers, there is no doubt what the verdict would have been, for there is no subject on which women feel with such passionate earnestness at the present time.

She continued by complaining that the specific interests of women were not taken seriously by the organisation:

> It is no new thing for the women of the Labour Party to find questions of particular interest to themselves placed at the end of a long agenda.[53]

This pattern continued. Throughout the decade the Organisation of Labour Women's policy in favour of birth control was constantly rejected by the Labour Party as a whole. Similarly, on the one occasion on which a Bill in favour of birth control was presented to the Commons (the Thurtle Ten Minute Bill) only 28 Labour MPs voted in favour while 46 voted against.[54] The women responded to this situation by unsuccessfully agitating for constitutional changes which would increase their strength in the organisation.[55]

Many historians have utilised an analysis of male power and attributed the persistent resistance to birth control within the Labour Party to gender conflict.[56] Although undoubtedly important, this is not an adequate explanation. The Party did not set out to marginalise the Organisation of Labour Women and ignore their wishes. This would have been quite foolhardy considering that by June 1921 it had between 60,000 and 80,000 members organised into about 620 women's sections.[57] In addition, Labour was very concerned to win over the new female voters.[58]

Throughout the decade, the male leadership did take the women's suggestions seriously on issues of which they approved. The most prominent area of cooperation was infant and maternal welfare, which both men and women members of the Labour Party considered to be the women's province. In this case, maternal welfare policy debated and adopted by the women, minus their calls for birth control, laid the basis for the development of Labour Party policy. The male leadership did not reject all the women's proposals but were determined not to concede on the particular issue of birth control. There is therefore a specific problem to be explained. A second point of great significance needs to be stressed: there was also great opposition to the birth control campaigners from the leadership of the Organisation of Labour Women. Throughout the 1920s there was a clear division between the leadership of the Organisation and the vast majority of the membership. The campaign would have been much more influential had it gained the support of leading Labour women. This lack of support was due to a clash of interests between their feminism and their socialism. The WBCG attempted to combine the two in their presentation of the needs of working-class women. Leading Labour women were not able to do so. They regarded the electoral opportunities of the Labour Party as the best chance for socialists to achieve their aims, and believed that controversial proposals, such as birth control, could only damage these. The battle lines were not simply gender-determined but related to the entire political philosophy of the Labour Party. (See also Chapter 7.)

Politics and parliamentarianism

The campaign for birth control raised a great deal of controversy because it brought questions concerning sexuality into the public political arena. The Labour Party was divided and afraid of losing possible votes, particularly from their Roman Catholic constituency. The leaderships of the Party and of the Organisation of Labour Women therefore found the whole question of birth control politically embarrassing. Throughout the 1920s there was very little discussion of the issue in the pages of *The Labour Woman*, despite continuous local activity and speaking tours organised by the campaigners. An editorial by Marion Phillips in March 1924 set the tone for the decade. She presented birth control as the antithesis of social reform and outlined the leadership's position. She stressed the lack of unanimity within the Labour Party and argued that because doctors and scientists disagreed over the desirability of birth control and the safety of various methods, more research was needed. In any case, sexual relations should not be regarded as a political issue. In the same year, Rose Witcop wrote to Margaret Sanger telling her that the birth control campaigners were under pressure in their local sections not to embarrass the Labour government.[59] There were therefore clear indications that, although individual members and branches had started becoming involved in the birth control campaign, the Party leadership considered the subject too controversial to adopt as party policy. A brief examination of the internal party debate confirms this proposition.

Those women who campaigned for birth control were consistently opposed by the leadership of their own organisation. The very first time the issue was raised at a conference of Labour Women in 1923 Dr Ethel Bentham, amidst protest, intervened in the debate. She argued that as the question was too complicated to be dealt with hurriedly at the end of the session it should be referred, with other resolutions, to the Standing Joint Committee.[60] Ethel Bentham was a member of the Labour Party Executive who was consistently opposed to birth control. In her autobiography, Dora Russell recounts an incident at the 1924 Women's Conference where she was confronted by Marion Phillips who told her to withdraw the addendum in favour of birth control, arguing against sex being dragged into politics.[61] The birth control addendum to the Report and Resolution on Maternity Care was not withdrawn and was passed overwhelmingly: 1,000 to 8. The entire report was then presented by a Standing Joint Committee Deputation to the Minister of Health, John Wheatley. On this occasion, instead of supporting the deputation, Marion Phillips 'suggested that there was more loose talk on birth control than on any other medical subject; it might well be the subject of an expert inquiry'. Wheatley, himself a Roman Catholic, agreed to this position.[62]

At the 1925 Conference of Labour Women, Frida Laski made a pointed reference to these divisions within the women's organisation:

[s]he was sure they would forgive her if she addressed what she had to say to the platform, because she believed the women in the audience were already committed.[63]

Within the Organisation of Labour Women this lack of support was consistently overcome as motions in favour of birth control were passed at consecutive conferences. This outcome was not repeated at Labour Party Conferences where leading Labour women played a crucial part in determining the fate of birth control resolutions. In a letter to *Labour Woman*, Dora Russell expressed dismay at the outcome of the 1925 Labour Party Conference at which the birth controllers were defeated:

> Without personal hostility to Mrs Harrison Bell, many of us were surprised that she supported the executive at Liverpool. Four seats are reserved for women on the National Executive. Why reserve seats for women at all, if they are not to represent the views of Labour Women?[64]

The WBCG persevered, pursuing a strategy of trying to win over the Labour Party, apparently successfully at the 1926 Party Conference. Dora Russell and Dorothy Jewson won a vote to reject the Executive's recommendation that birth control should not be made a party political issue. However, later in the Conference the Standing Orders Committee announced that, after consultation with the Executive, they had decided that 'the vote recorded did not commit the Party on the principle involved, and that the whole question be referred to the new Executive Committee for consideration and report to the next Conference'. This was agreed to by the Conference.[65] These two votes were obviously highly contradictory. The first vote was the only defeat recorded against the Executive's views at the Conference and was a result of the consistent activity of the WBCG which had succeeded in gaining the votes of the – mainly male – Conference delegates. The second vote was a significant victory for the leadership in their immediate quest to nullify the first.

At this stage national political developments played a significant part in the birth control campaign. Large sections of the Labour movement had acted independently of the Labour Party leadership during the General Strike and the miners' lockout. This activity, combined with an acknowledgement of the vital supporting role played by women, undoubtedly contributed to the WBCG's initial victory at the Labour Party Conference in 1926. They had gained the votes of many trade union delegates, including the miners' contingent. By the following year the mood was very different. The defeat of the General Strike and of the miners, combined with the proximity of a general election, ensured that the Labour Party's vision of socialism through parliamentary methods had gained hegemony within the Labour movement. The trade unions now looked towards the Party to achieve through parliamentary means what they had failed to achieve through industrial struggle. The conflict between socialism and feminism also became more acute. As the general election loomed ever nearer the resolve of the women's organisation weakened. The women's leadership became more concerned to support the Labour Party Executive and their arguments found greater resonance within the Organisation of Labour Women.

The Labour Party leadership very quickly regained control over the birth control issue. The Executive's recommendation in the Party's 1927 Annual Report was, once again, that the issue should not become party political. This position was openly supported by Marion Phillips.[66] At the 1927 Party Conference the Executive were determined to win: they enlisted the support of several women,[67] who spoke against the birth controllers, and Arthur Henderson delivered a telling speech, later printed in full in *The Labour Woman*. He made quite clear his belief that Labour's victory in the forthcoming election was at stake:

> If the recommendation was turned down what would be the position in the months that were before them, when they were preparing for what might be the most important election that the Party had ever known?[68]

The vote of 2,885,000 to 275,000 spelt the final defeat of the WBCG's attempt to convince the Labour Party to adopt a favourable policy towards improving the provision of birth control.

The Executive were not content with this outcome. The following year they turned their attention to winning their position on birth control at the Conference of Labour Women. For the first time a male member of the Executive attended to speak on birth control. Arthur Henderson was supported by Ellen Wilkinson and by 273 to 270 they won the vote deciding that birth control should not be a party political issue. This was a significant defeat for the birth control campaigners: Labour Women had fallen in behind the Labour Party Executive. The fact that Ellen Wilkinson, a well-known campaigner for working women's rights, took a public position against the birth control campaigners is significant, and has puzzled historians who have assumed that she did not support the campaign.[69] This was not the case: private letters from Wilkinson to Dora Russell in May 1930 demonstrate that she supported the birth control campaigners and was working for the ban to be lifted.[70] The fact that the Executive were able to enlist her support in defeating the birth control campaigners at the women's conference is a clear indication that, in public, leading women were being forced to choose between their socialism and their feminism.

This failure revealed the weakness of the WBCG's political strategy. They sought to commit a future Labour government to a policy in favour of distributing birth control information, but the Party leadership believed that an election victory was inconceivable with such a controversial proposal adopted as Party policy. In 1928 Labour Party women finally sacrificed their own desires in favour of electoral considerations. The shortcomings of this parliamentary approach were also highlighted by the relative success of the WBCG's campaigning activity at a local level.

The local authority campaign

The WBCG had enjoyed considerable local support, and organised local activity, since its formation. Local campaigners had been responsible for maintaining steady pressure on local health authorities to take initiatives regarding birth control provision. Towards the end of the decade this activity was given greater importance in its own right, and paid dividends. While the 1928 defeat illustrated the control of the leadership over the Labour Party machine, the success of the local campaign was a genuine reflection of the strength of support for birth control at a rank and file level in the Labour movement. The WBCG were able to include a positive approach towards birth control within their proposals concerning the needs of working-class women as 'consumers' of welfare. In many cases, Labour women were able to influence local government policy on infant and maternal welfare through holding positions as local councillors and on advisory committees. The WBCG's local campaign consciously aimed at local authorities in their role as providers of infant and maternal welfare.

Campaigning activity comprised successive speaking tours, local petitions and resolutions, and constant correspondence with local health authorities. There was a bout of activity in 1926 which resulted in the Ministry of Health being inundated with resolutions from local authorities. As efforts to change Labour Party policy were faltering, this local activity began to show results. In 1929 the campaign picked up again. Local meetings and campaigns were organised to coincide with formal resolutions, in favour of birth control, being raised in local councils. By 7 February 1930, only two months after Shoreditch had passed the first resolution, fifty-five local authorities had sent resolutions to the Minister of Health asking him

> [t]o give consideration to the question of allowing municipalities to provide facilities for reliable and private information as to the methods of family limitation.[71]

In addition, some local authorities took the step of going ahead and giving birth control advice without official sanction. This was partly prompted by the 1929 Local Government Act which expanded the powers of local officials and helped to remove their fear of losing government grants.[72] This local activity culminated in a large *Conference on the Giving of Information on Birth Control by Public Health Authorities* on 4 April 1930.[73] This Conference, attended by delegates from thirty-five public health authorities, sixteen maternal and child welfare centres and 132 other organisations, forwarded a resolution to the Minister of Health. It undoubtedly strengthened the resolve of local authorities to permit the provision of birth control information. By July 1930, when the Ministry of Health finally reversed its policy, it was very much a case of officially permitting local authorities to do what a growing and visible number of them were already doing.

CONCLUSION

In 1930, under the new Labour administration, the Ministry of Health issued Memorandum 153/MCW. This authorised local authorities to permit birth control advice for medical reasons. By restricting its application to medical cases only, they had attempted to ensure that the least number of people could possibly be offended while conceding the minimum demand of the campaigners. The policy was a compromise. The Ministry quite specifically rejected any possibility of granting birth control on request, thereby denying women the opportunity to control their own fertility. The basis was laid for the policy of family planning under the control of the medical profession.

It is important, however, not to read this history through the ideology of second-wave feminism. This reform was also precisely what the campaigners had fought for. The WBCG's main concern was to increase the status and care of mothers rather than challenging gender relations. Without moving out of this maternal feminism the transformation of the social relations of reproduction that later feminists looked for could not take place. The campaigners did not demand an end to the sexual division of labour but what they achieved laid the basis for any future challenge to that division of labour.

A measure of the scale of the victory is that even the WBCG's moderate approach was not enough for birth control to be accepted without a massive struggle. In this struggle they enjoyed great success at a local level where Labour movement women focused on the question of maternal health, and were able to exert influence over the provision of local services. At the national level, anxieties connected with competing ideologies of sexuality and gender relations intruded and electoral considerations prevailed. In this respect it is significant that the concession was finally wrung from a Labour administration in a post- rather than a pre-election period. The whole question of women's control of their fertility and of their sexuality was inevitably part of the campaign. It was this element that signified the campaigners' challenge to many of the existing ideas in the 1920s, and it was this that made their victory a vital step in the struggle to break the bond between sex and reproduction.

NOTES

1 Cited in E. How-Martyn and M. Breed, *The Birth Control Movement in Britain*, London, John Bale, Sons & Danielson Ltd, 1930, p. 26.
2 This chapter is intended as a contribution to the debate on this particular campaign in the 1920s. The material presented is based upon archive research into the Organisation of Labour Women and the Workers' Birth Control Group. The Organisation of Labour Women's archives are located in the Labour Party libraries at Walworth Road, London, and in Manchester. Archives for the WBCG were difficult to locate and much of the information in this chapter was gathered from the Dora Russell Papers at the International Institute of Social History (IISH) in Amsterdam. Dora Russell was the Secretary of the WBCG for most of the period under investigation.
3 N. and V. Himes, 'Birth Control for the British Working Class', *Hospital Social Service*, 1929, vol. 19, p. 580.
4 Audrey Leathard, *The Fight for Family Planning*, London, Macmillan, 1980; How-Martyn and Breed, *Birth Control Movement*; Richard Soloway, *Birth Control and the Population Question in England*, London, Chapel Hill, 1982.

5 Memorandum 153/MCW was agreed by the Cabinet in July 1930 but only officially printed and issued by HMSO in 1931.

6 Leathard, *Fight for Family Planning*, is a thorough history of the Family Planning Association which concentrates on the development of the voluntary clinics. Both R. Ledbetter, *A History of the Malthusian League: 1877–1927*, Columbus, Ohio State University Press, 1976, and Miriam J. Benn, *The Predicaments of Love*, London, Pluto Press, 1992, concentrate exclusively on the Malthusian League. The two most authoritative biographies of Marie Stopes (Ruth Hall, *Marie Stopes: A Biography*, London, Andre Deutsch, 1977, and June Rose, *Marie Stopes and the Sexual Revolution*, London, Faber & Faber, 1992) do not stray beyond their remits. The more political campaign, involving working-class women, which tried to persuade successive governments to change policy, has only been touched upon in a number of works. L. Ward, *The Right to Choose: A Study of Women's Fight for Birth Control Provisions*, University of Bristol, unpublished PhD thesis, 1981, does analyse the political campaign in some detail but her discussion of the WBCG suffers from limited access to material. In addition, Ward's emphasis on birth control as a feminist issue causes her to underestimate the class aspect of the campaign in the 1920s. Ward also discusses the important part played by the Women's Co-operative Guild in the campaign in the 1920s.

7 In order to clarify differences in approach between feminism and socialism I have adopted simple working definitions. These are to view socialism as a political movement to transform society on egalitarian principles to the benefit of the working class, and feminism as a political movement to overcome inequalities between the sexes. Within these definitions there is obviously room for a wide variety of approaches. In the 1920s there was no political current that called itself socialist-feminist but there were women who tried to combine a commitment to both ideals in their political activity.

8 Leathard, *Fight for Family Planning*; Sheila Rowbotham, *A New World for Women: Stella Browne: Socialist Feminist*, London, Pluto Press, 1977; Ward, *Right to Choose*. Pamela Graves, *Labour Women: Women in British Working Class Politics*, Cambridge, Cambridge University Press, 1994, takes into consideration the political priorities of the Labour Party in the 1920s but still ends with attributing the resistance to different gender priorities.

9 WBCG, *Objects*, London, WBCG, 1927.

10 Dora Russell, *Report on the Founding and Work of the Workers' Birth Control Group and the Attitude of the English Labour Party towards Birth Control*, London, WBCG, 1925, p. 5.

11 Hall, *Marie Stopes*, and Rose, *Marie Stopes*, concur in this general assessment. June Rose lays greater stress on Stopes' promotion of birth control as one aspect of her espousal of radical ideas on sexuality, while Ruth Hall is generally more critical, emphasising Stopes' proposals for eugenically inspired population policies and even linking her ideas to those of Hitler. Although eugenic ideas did cross the political spectrum, the extent to which they were

compatible with progressive thought is much disputed. See Michael Freeden, 'Eugenics and Progressive Thought: A Study in Ideological Affinity', *Historical Journal*, 1979, vol. 22, no. 3, pp. 645–71 and Greta Jones, 'Eugenics and Social Policy between the Wars', *Historical Journal*, 1982, vol. 25, no. 3, pp. 717–28. What cannot be disputed is that the eugenic ideas of Marie Stopes were thoroughly conservative.

12 Benn, *Predicaments of Love*, and Ledbetter, *Malthusian League*, make it clear that in the 1920s the League clung to the tenet that the solution to poverty was to curtail the breeding of the poorer classes. See N. Haire, *Hygienic Methods of Family Limitation*, London, Malthusian League, 1922; E. Daniels, *The Children of Desire*, London, E. Daniels, 1925; and T. Stewart, *The Case for Birth Control or Neo-Malthusianism*, London, The Freedom League, 1923, for examples of the League's political approach in the 1920s.
13 Dora Russell, *The Tamarisk Tree: Volume One*, London, Virago, 1977, p. 173.
14 *The Labour Woman*, May 1924, p. 80.
15 *The Labour Woman*, November 1926, pp. 167–8.
16 Francois Bédarida, *A Social History of England 1851–1975*, London, Methuen, 1979.
17 Robert Dowse, *Left in the Centre: The Independent Labour Party 1893–1940*, London, Longman, 1966.
18 Graves, *Labour Women*; Lucy Middleton (ed.), *Women in the Labour Movement*, London, Croom Helm, 1977; Vicky Randall, *Women and Politics*, London, Macmillan, 1987; Sheila Rowbotham and Jeffrey Weeks, *Socialism and the New Life*, London, Pluto Press, 1977. See Vera Brittain, *Testament of Youth*, London, Fontana, 1979, for a personal account.
19 See Dorothy Jewson, *Socialists and the Family*, London, ILP, 1926; and M. Pallister, *Socialism for Women*, London, ILP, 1924.
20 WBCG, *Memorandum on the Question of Birth Control*, London, WBCG, 1924.
21 WBCG, *Memorandum on Maternity Care*, London, WBCG, 1925.
22 WBCG, *Objects*.
23 The Labour Party, *Twenty Sixth Annual Report of the Labour Party*, London, the Labour Party, 1926, p. 202.
24 *Twenty Seventh Annual Report of the Labour Party*, p. 233.
25 *Parliamentary Debates*, 5th Series, 1924, vol. 176, col. 2050.
26 WBCG, *Memorandum on Birth Control*.
27 *The Labour Woman*, 1 June 1924, p. 96.
28 Olive Banks, *Faces of Feminism*, Oxford, Basil Blackwell, 1986; Rowbotham, *New World for Women*; F. Williams, *Social Policy: A Critical Introduction*, Oxford, Polity Press, 1989.
29 Margaret Llewelyn Davies (ed.), *Maternity: Letters from Working Women*, London, Virago, 1978; S. Ferguson, 'Labour Women and the Social Services', in Middleton (ed.), *Women in the Labour Movement*; Pat Thane, 'Visions of Gender in the Making of the British Welfare State: the Case of Women in the British Labour Party and Social Policy, 1906–1945', in Gisella Bock and Pat Thane (eds), *Maternity*

and Gender Policies: Women and the Rise of the European Welfare States 1880s–1950s, London, Routledge, 1991.
30 Jane Lewis, *Women in England: 1870–1950*, Sussex, Wheatsheaf Books, 1984. See also Diana Gittins, *Fair Sex: Family Size and Structure*, London, Hutchinson, 1982 and Jane Lewis, *The Politics of Motherhood*, London, Croom Helm, 1980.
31 Rowbotham, *New World for Women.*
32 Thane, 'Visions of Gender.'
33 Russell, *Report.*
34 Circular dated April 1924, Dora Russell Papers, IISH, Amsterdam.
35 Russell, *Report.*
36 Russell, *Report*, p. 6.
37 Rowbotham, *New World for Women.*
38 Letter from Stella Browne to Dora Russell 5/11/1923. Dora Russell Papers, IISH, Amsterdam.
39 WBCG, *Memorandum on Birth Control*, p. 3.
40 Linda Gordon, *Woman's Body, Woman's Right*, Middlesex, Penguin, 1977.
41 Russell, *Tamarisk Tree*, p. 176.
42 Carol Dyhouse, *Feminism and the Family in England 1880–1939*, Oxford, Basil Blackwell, 1989; Randall, *Women and Politics*; Jeffrey Weeks, *Sexuality*, London, Tavistock, 1986.
43 Ronald Blythe, *The Age of Illusion: England in the Twenties and Thirties*, London, Hamish Hamilton, 1963.
44 Mary Scharlieb, *Artificial Limitation of the Birth-Rate*, London, Putnams, n.d., p. 6.
45 Dora Russell Papers, IISH, Amsterdam.
46 *The Labour Woman*, June 1923, p. 99.
47 Dora Russell was also concerned to maintain a respectable distance from the campaign for abortion law reform which she feared could damage the WBCG's cause: Russell, *Tamarisk Tree.*
48 Dora Russell Papers, IISH, Amsterdam.
49 WBCG, *Memorandum on Birth Control*, pp. 7–8.
50 WBCG, *Medical Views on Birth Control*, London, WBCG, 1925.
51 Dora Russell letter to *Socialist Review*, May 1925.
52 Graves, *Labour Women.*
53 'The New Generation', quoted in Rowbotham, *New World for Women*, p. 35.
54 *Parliamentary Debates*, 5th Series, 1926, vol. 191, cols 849-85.
55 Graves, *Labour Women.*
56 See note 8.
57 *The Labour Woman*, June 1921, p. 98.
58 Graves, *Labour Women*, estimates that an expected five million working-class women were due to be enfranchised.
59 Soloway, *Birth Control*, p. 286.
60 The Organisation of Labour Women was directed by the Standing Joint Committee of Industrial Women's Organisations (SJC), which was an Advisory Committee to the Executive of the Labour Party.
61 Russell, *Tamarisk Tree*, p. 172.

62 *The Labour Woman*, September 1924, p. 145. In May 1924 Wheatley had summarily rejected a previous deputation and petition in favour of birth control.

63 *The Labour Woman*, August 1925, p. 213.

64 *The Labour Woman*, December 1925, p. 206.

65 *The Labour Woman*, November 1926, p. 167.

66 *The Labour Woman*, October 1927, p. 146.

67 Miss Quinn, Mrs Redgrave and Dr Stella Churchill.

68 *The Labour Woman*, October 1927, p. 167.

69 Betty Vernon, *Ellen Wilkinson*, London, Croom Helm, 1982; and Graves, *Labour Women*.

70 Dora Russell Papers, IISH, Amsterdam.

71 *Parliamentary Debates,* 5th Series, 1930, vol. 324, col.1174.

72 Soloway, *Birth Control*; Ward, *Right to Choose*.

73 Report, *Conference on the Giving of Information on Birth Control by Public Health Authorities*, 1930. The conference was organised by The National Union of Societies for Equal Citizenship, The Society for the Provision of Birth Control Clinics, The Women's National Liberal Federation and the Worker's Birth Control Group.

Chapter 7

'The children's party, therefore the women's party'

The Labour Party and child welfare in inter-war Britain[1]

John Stewart

The Labour Party was, from its foundation in 1900, concerned with child welfare. In the inter-war period, one of the many illustrations of this can be found in 1929 in *Children First!*, wherein Labour described itself as 'the party of childhood, because it is the party of the future. It is the trustee of the nation of tomorrow.' Consequently, Labour's child welfare policies were 'directed to that most important of political aims, making the world safe for the coming generation'. Such attitudes might be seen as being summed up by two publications in 1937. The significantly titled *Children's Charter*, produced by Labour women, proposed a range of solutions to the problems apparently facing British children. More succinctly, the National Campaign Committee brought out a poster with the heading 'Children – The Pride of the Nation'.[2] Why did Labour emphasise child welfare? It would be wrong to argue that it was the only party concerned with such matters. The 1920s and 1930s saw, for example, the growth of the movements for family allowances and for better infant welfare provision, both supported by individuals and organisations across the political spectrum. Nonetheless Labour clearly saw itself as both especially concerned with children, and uniquely qualified to be so. It was quick to acknowledge the significance of already-existing child welfare provision, and anxious to see these expanded and new services introduced: as G. D. H. Cole put it in respect of school medical services in 1924, 'what has been accomplished only serves to emphasise the need for fuller provisions'.[3]

The reasons for this attitude are the subject of this chapter. It will be argued that gender was significant for at least two reasons. First, child welfare was seen as having the potential to capture a large part of the women's vote, at both national and local level, thereby appealing to women as 'consumers' of welfare. Second, Labour movement women were active in promoting child welfare measures – in this capacity acting as potential or actual 'providers'. However, it will also be suggested that, for Labour, child welfare was more than simply a gender issue. Nutritional standards, for example, were important, particularly in an era of intense economic depression. Any further decline in child health was deemed potentially disastrous for both the already beleaguered Labour movement and the nation as a whole. Despite these concerns, however, the Labour leadership was unwilling to commit itself to any clear and coherent programme of child welfare. This resulted from an inability to balance the demands of economic recovery with those of social policy; and from the nature of the relationship between the Labour leadership and bodies such as its women's organisations. (See also Chapter 6.) Child welfare therefore clearly illustrates the Labour Party's problems in formulating health and welfare policy in a crucial era in its history and in welfare development.

I have suggested elsewhere that before 1914 Labour concern for child welfare was motivated by humanitarianism; by labour market issues; by the view of healthy children as the future creators and beneficiaries of a socialist society; and by more general fears over 'racial health'. For Labour, welfare targeted at children was to take place within a family context, the stable working-class family being a model for a future socialist society. The idea of direct state control of children was rejected, although it was acknowledged that both the community and children themselves had rights which might, on occasion, transcend the family's. This analysis of children's welfare needs, therefore, contributed to the Labour Party's attempt to define, in its own terms, that most elusive of concepts, 'socialism'.[4]

Pre-war attitudes persisted after 1918. Philip Snowden described infant mortality as an 'incalculable social loss', and emphasised the importance of ensuring that children's bodies and minds were catered for. Attempts to educate children 'ill-fed, ill-nourished and suffering from diseases' wasted time and resources, hence the need for greater medical provision. A Party report of 1921 asserted that economically nothing could be more important than 'to gain better conditions for (children)', while in 1937 Mary Sutherland, the Chief Woman Officer, was at pains to deny Tory claims that extending the school meals service would undermine parental responsibility and thereby family life. And, as the official Labour Party obituary of the child welfare campaigner Margaret McMillan put it, 'if Socialism is to be achieved ... by a healthy and educated democracy, the influences that surround and mould the earlier years of working class children must be potent for progress'.[5] So continuities existed between pre- and post-World War I concerns. But while the general outlines remained similar, there were also important differences and developments. Political circumstances had changed; a more 'scientific' approach to health was developing; and the question of how to provide and organise social welfare had taken on greater urgency, not least because of the conflicting claims of fiscal responsibility and widespread social distress. The condition of the nation's children therefore continued to be of concern to the Labour movement, although precisely what to do about it was rather more problematical.

WOMEN AND CHILD WELFARE

Among the most obvious political changes of the post-war era was the gaining of the parliamentary franchise by women, partially in 1918 and fully in 1928. A 1921 Labour Party report felt the 'protection of motherhood and infancy and the nurture of children' were 'political questions of primary importance', not least because of 'the power which women have acquired'.[6] Labour was in competition with other political parties for these new voters. Its main rival after 1918, the Conservative Party, also adapted its message to new circumstances, and did so in part by emphasising its role, locally and nationally, in providing child welfare. But the Conservatives also preached the message of domestic economy as a metaphor for national economy at a time when, as Labour propagandists endlessly pointed out, child welfare provision was being cut.[7] Just as Labour put itself forward as uniquely concerned with childhood, so too did it emphasise that, in such a context, it was also naturally the party of women. It did so by presenting itself as deeply committed to social welfare and, in particular, to child welfare.

More pragmatically, women were potential 'consumers' of child welfare, and Labour's appeal to women on this basis was seen as reaping clear rewards. Andrew Young MP attributed his 1924 election victory to 'the cry of the children. I won the hearts of the mothers, and that . . . was how I won Partick.' In 1929 *Women and the General Election* argued that women's admission to the political process had made the child the 'central figure'. Any sense of progress or 'perfectibility' depended on creating the proper environment for child development, and so 'the effect of any measure on the nation's children is the test, the touchstone of its value'.[8] Clearly, it was felt that women and children were linked, and that this could work to Labour's electoral advantage.

Child welfare issues were also heavily concentrated upon by Labour women themselves. The Standing Joint Committee of Industrial Women's Organisations (SJCIWO), for example, presented a memorandum on nursery education to the Board of Education in 1932. The organisation's chair, Barbara Ayrton Gould, stressed its medical and educational benefits, and saw it as a 'special aim' of women to demand nursery provision, so that the effects of depression and poverty might be ameliorated.[9] Labour women were, therefore, undoubtedly concerned with child welfare. But this was not unproblematical. There was an ambiguous relationship between the women's organisations and the national leadership. One instance of this came in 1927, when Ramsay MacDonald found it 'undesirable' that a matter of policy, in this case family allowances, be discussed at women's conference. Far better, he felt, that a general discussion take place which would of its nature be non-committal.[10] Furthermore, Labour women could be divided not on the issue of increased child welfare provision – which all Labour women, and indeed most Labour men, agreed with – but rather on the form it should take.

The case of family allowances

This was especially clear regarding the contentious issue of cash family allowances. *The Labour Woman* noted among its readers a 'very strong feeling' in their favour. Similarly, some women prominent in the Labour movement, such as Averil Furniss, saw cash family allowances as important in furthering female emancipation. But others held markedly different views. As early as 1923 the female proposer of a conference motion on 'Motherhood and Child Endowment' argued for payments in kind, as cash payments would simply lead to price inflation. Dr Marion Phillips, the party's principal women's officer, told the TUC and Labour Party Joint Committee on Family Allowances that 'there is not a great deal of interest in Family Endowment in the country'. Of more concern were 'practical steps to make child welfare a reality, in the development of maternity services and in education'. A Co-operative movement witness expressed similar views. Nor did Phillips feel cash allowances to be particularly important to working women in respect of sexual equality. There were therefore divisions within Labour women over family allowances. These were heightened by the scepticism of many about the leading proponent of family allowances, Eleanor Rathbone, who was felt to be out of touch with working-class living conditions. This points to class divisions between working-class and middle-class women over cash allowances.[11]

Indeed the issue of family allowances provides a useful insight into how various factors – gender, class, professional knowledge – could intersect in the formation of welfare policy. It is well known that the majority report of the Labour movement committee, which recommended cash allowances, was rejected by the TUC. In its place the minority report, which was much more sceptical about cash allowances, was endorsed. In terms of the relationship between party and unions it was significant that Labour, despite pressure from the Independent Labour Party (ILP) and a number of its local organisations, was at pains to await TUC deliberation on the matter. The TUC's decision, which shaped the Labour movement's official attitude to family allowances throughout the 1930s, is usually put down to union fears over the impact of cash benefits on collective bargaining. Clearly there is much to this argument.[12] However, the matter is more than simply one of narrow union 'economism'.

The minority report noted the scepticism of the Labour MP and London County Council (LCC) member, Dr Alfred Salter, as to the efficacy of allocating welfare resources to cash allowances. Much to be preferred were 'collective schemes for health and education services'. Salter, in his evidence to the TUC/Labour Party Joint Committee, had been critical of cash allowances, suggesting that even were such a large sum as £130 million available it would 'be better spent on social services than on Family Allowances'. His doubts were shared by his socialist medical colleague, Somerville Hastings. In a debate with a cash family allowances proponent, the ILP's Jennie Lee, Hastings affirmed his belief that it was beyond question that children were the nation's 'most valuable asset'. Money had to be spent on them. But what was important was collective rather than individual allocation. The former would be more efficient and, significantly, cheaper. Fiscal responsibility was important, and much concern on this topic had been expressed by the minority report and the TUC/Labour Party Joint Committee, not least because of the other social service commitments.

But on another level Hastings was also making an important point about the provision of child welfare. Were cash to be given to the mother, he suggested, it might be spent on nutritionally inferior food. Better, therefore, to allocate resources to a state medical service which would, at no cost to the parents, provide children with all they required. These points, particularly that concerning the inadequate knowledge of mothers, had been made by both Hastings and Salter to the Joint Committee.[13] Unsurprisingly, Hastings was criticised for this approach, one correspondent to *The Labour Woman* exclaiming: 'Oh! the mentality of men, especially of those who are not fathers of working class families. One wonders how much some of our MPs do understand of the management and economy of a working class home'. This was a fair point, but the very scale of child poverty in this period clearly influenced commentators such as Hastings. Furthermore, the idea of collective rather than individual social provision raises important issues about how welfare resources should be allocated, and the role of 'specialist' knowledge in so doing.[14] The socio-economic context of inter-war Britain also needs to be borne in mind. The Labour movement was, for most of the period, on the defensive. It appears to have been suspicious of strictly monetary welfare benefits such as cash family allowances, partly because of their perceived impact on wages, but also because they could be relatively easily withdrawn. It was therefore desirable to have institutions, such as collective child health services, which were easier to defend. Such services would be seen as a 'right' rather than a matter of 'largesse'. On a more practical level, British labour was certainly aware of the development of family allowance schemes in Europe, which at least in the early 1920s appeared not always to operate to the benefit of organised labour.[15]

The collective welfare provision advocated by health professionals such as Salter and Hastings was influential in Labour movement child welfare debates. Collectivist arguments were used during the TUC debate on family allowances and by the TUC delegate, George Gibson, to the British Medical Association's (BMA) 1939 Nutrition Conference. Gibson certainly emphasised TUC apprehension about the potential impact of cash family allowances on wage negotiations. But he also argued for a full and comprehensive health service for children, covering both prevention and treatment from birth to school-leaving age, and for other measures to improve the condition of child life. Similarly, he questioned whether 'the average parent of the middle class, let alone the working classes, is competent to decide the best method of allotting an increased income in respect of the absolute welfare and future outlook of a child'. For the benefit of the children and for the nation's future child welfare had to be recognised as a national responsibility, and one to be dealt with collectively.[16] It was also significant that cash allowances were rejected in the *Children's Charter*. This suggested that nobody doubted the 'special responsibility' of mothers for child well-being. But many of the needs of children could be 'better ... met by the community than by the individual home – and this would still be true even if the burden of extreme poverty were lifted from the thousands of homes overshadowed by this burden today'.[17]

The debate over cash family allowances therefore provides crucial insights to gender concerns and gender relationships within the Labour movement. But it must also be recognised that it manifested a profound, if not yet clearly articulated, concern over the nature of any future welfare provision. Pedersen is right to emphasise the central role of male wage concerns over the matter of cash allowances, but is perhaps over-dismissive of the impact of other arguments, especially that on health provision. However, the newly enfranchised woman was a key component in shaping Labour's approach to child welfare, and Thane has recently pointed to the influence of Labour women in structuring British welfare provision, not least in local bodies.[18]

The significance of local politics

This in turn suggests that local politics was important in the agitation for improved child welfare. At parliamentary level Labour had limited success in the inter-war period, and after 1931 there seemed little immediate hope of forming another government. Local government was another matter, and important for child welfare because the bulk of existing provision was the responsibility of local bodies – a point made forcefully by, among others, Beatrice Webb. Moreover, the issue of child welfare was clearly perceived as an important local political weapon in its own right. The 'Educational Programme for Local Councillors' put forward in *The Labour Woman* in 1925 emphasised the need for free medical inspection and treatment, school meals, and more general improvements in the school environment. In 1929 Susan Lawrence, under-secretary at the Ministry of Health, stressed the importance of municipal control if health problems such as child mortality were to be brought under control and pointed to the difference in health conditions between different parts of the country.[19] Such regional variations were picked up, sometimes rather crudely, in Labour propaganda. The 1928 leaflet *Preserve the Real Wealth of the Nation*, namely children, listed the infant mortality rates for four areas: Battersea, Woolwich, Wigan and South Shields. As was made clear, the first two had Labour councils and low infant mortality rates, the last two had neither. On the whole, Labour tended not to accuse its political opponents of actually murdering children, most propaganda leaving it to readers to draw their own conclusions. Once again, much of the relevant literature appears to have been directed at women.[20]

More positively, Fenner Brockway claimed significant child health improvements in Labour Bermondsey in the 1920s while H. R. S. Phillpott, in his 1934 survey of Labour authorities, pointed to the maternity and child welfare services now provided in Lincoln and to the growth of school meal provision in Durham. Labour clearly took local provision of child welfare extremely seriously, providing their potential and actual representatives with twelve pages of statistical material in 1938, and claiming in a leaflet of the same year that 'Your Councillors have a great responsibility towards the children – the citizens of the future'. Indeed the mid- to late 1930s saw a Labour push in local politics and a realisation that health matters, especially those concerning children, were politically significant. This relationship is borne out in a letter from the party's local government department to the Socialist Medical Association (SMA) stressing the growth of local government activity and the 'real need for pamphlets on nutrition, state hospitals, and the development of the maternity and child welfare services'.[21] Labour's most spectacular local success in the inter-war period was its capture of the London County Council in 1934. Although a deeply cautious body, the Labour

LCC did make progress in child welfare provision, particularly in areas such as school meals and medical inspection.[22]

THE NATION'S FUTURE

So political concerns, based on the changed post-war electorate and the demands of local politics, played a significant part in Labour's approach to child welfare. There was also a wider view. At a rather sentimental level, but one which combined an appeal to women with broader issues, it was claimed in 1937 that 'Baby is his mother's most precious possession. Britain's babies are Britain's most precious possession.' With the growth of fascism and international tension in the 1930s the relationship between the future of the nation and children's mental and physical condition became more clearly articulated. In 1935 Katharine Bruce Glasier related that the two most popular themes on her recent speaking tour had been 'The Road to Peace on Earth' and 'The Battle for Our Children's Lives'. She found this unsurprising as women had always known the two to be related. The battles against militarism and poverty were 'in reality one', not least because expenditure on arms could be more usefully employed on social services.[23]

But the issue was more complex still. Mary Sutherland, addressing Labour women in 1936, found underfeeding 'not only a question of physical health but mental health as well'. Might it not be, she suggested, that 'Hitler marched to power on the unbalanced nerves of a generation that was improperly fed and underfed as it grew up during the war and early post-war years'. This was an inter-war version of the established socialist belief that healthy children were the key to the advent of socialism; conversely, poorly nourished children were potentially a threat to democracy. The concern with direct action on child welfare also, in this context, led most on the political left to ridicule the national government's physical fitness campaign of the late 1930s. Labour MPs argued in the Commons during the passage of the 1937 Physical Training and Recreation Act that adequate nutrition had to precede physical education. Others in the Labour movement questioned the ends to which non-socialists propagated ideas of national health. Lucy Noel-Buxton saw the question of national health as an 'engrossing' one across the political spectrum, but suggested that only Labour approached this in a 'scientific' way and for reasons of national and international health. By contrast, the dictatorships, and indeed British Conservatives, were 'chiefly interested that their own nation should be healthy, so that it may win the war, if and when war comes'. Given official attitudes to, for example, physical education, this is not as unlikely as it might at first appear. As Welshman points out, plans for British schools in the late 1930s were heavily influenced by contemporary international rivalries. Child health and international affairs were not, therefore, separate issues, but intimately linked.[24]

Children and malnutrition

This concern about the role of children in securing the nation's future in an ever more unstable and complex world was further focused by concern about the nature and extent of malnutrition. Increasing in intensity in the 1930s with the expansion of international tension, economic depression, the growth of nutritional science, and the debate over physical training, this became extremely important to Labour's analysis of child welfare. Opening a Commons debate on malnutrition in 1936, the Labour MP Thomas Johnston claimed that 'other than the question of peace and war there is no graver issue that can be discussed by this Parliament'. The Labour movement had long argued that malnourishment and undernourishment existed. But the apparent scientific 'proofs' of the 1930s gave, as the 1935 NEC Report put it, 'a justification of the Party's Socialist policy', particularly at a time of escalating unemployment and of social service cuts.[25]

Why were children so central to Labour's concern over malnutrition? First, the very scale of child poverty was commented on by virtually all the inter-war social surveys, and was thereby almost impossible to ignore. Second, it was argued that ill-health in childhood would almost inevitably lead to ill-health in adulthood, and that this was effectively irreversible. This in turn would raise the threat of economic 'inefficiency', children frequently being referred to as the nation's 'capital'; and, as suggested earlier, the possibility that ill-developed minds could be seduced by irrationalist and anti-democratic politics. Third, it was claimed that working-class children were in a markedly poorer condition than their counterparts from other social groups and that this in itself was an indictment of capitalism. Ellen Wilkinson neatly made this point when, reviewing the existing data on child health, she concluded that 'good health is becoming a class question'.[26] Fourth, there was a considerable amount of data, however imperfect, available on child health. Once the problems which this revealed were fully recognised, steps could be taken to rectify them. Children were accessible to such solutions in that they were institutionalised, most obviously in schools, and there was also an existing network of care – school meals, maternity and child welfare centres, and so on – which, with political will, could be extended. Labour's emphasis on local politics is once again important here, although the party had no doubt that parliamentary power was necessary to fully implement its plans. As Hugh Dalton put it, what was required was a national health scheme, 'closely ... linked with the schools'. Hence the need for more systematic medical inspection and treatment alongside better provision of school meals and milk.[27]

As noted, Labour was never shy about indicting Coalition, Conservative or National governments for the poor state of the nation's children. In the early 1920s *The Labour Woman* urged its readers to 'Save the Children from Hunger!'. In the name of economy, the Provision of Meals Act was being attacked. This was 'frankly a policy of hunger'. Even as World War I – a period which had seen an expansion of child welfare services – came to an end, such themes were embryonically present. This suggests that pre-war Labour fears about child health, mental and physical, had not been allayed by wartime measures. Indeed a conference delegate in 1919 claimed that it was children who had made the greatest sacrifices during the war.[28] By the mid-1920s the themes of government betrayal, class difference and the implications of an ill-nourished child population were well in place. A joint TUC/Labour Party memorandum of 1922 noted that although scientific precision in these matters was not yet available, there could be 'no doubt the effects are disastrous'.[29] Labour propaganda and agitation in this period, although possibly effective in its own terms, nonetheless remained rather crude, a series of assertions rather indiscriminately blaming the government and/or capitalism for the woes of the nation's children.

By 1929, however, matters were becoming more sophisticated. A leaflet of that year asked: *The Health of the Nation: Why Are We C.3?* The answer, it was felt, was the poor state of public health and particularly that affecting children. Labour, it emphasised, 'Led the Way in Child Welfare', and among the proposals for a better state of national health were the development of the school medical service and nation-wide coverage of maternity and child welfare services. 'Vote For Labour', it concluded, 'And An A.1 Nation.' Or, as *Children First!* put it in the same year, '(Labour) holds that money spent in producing an A.1 generation is the soundest form of national investment'. By 1935 the Labour Party was laying the blame for poor public health clearly on the National Government which had, for example, cut back on school meals provision and discouraged nursery schools and maternal and child welfare. Once again, the advice to the electorate was to 'Vote Labour for an A.1 Nation'.[30] This classificatory, pseudo-scientific language was by no means new, but the frequency and intensity of its use increased as Labour, after the fall of the 1929–31 government, sought to show how malnourished working-class children were, especially those whose parents were unemployed and lived in areas of maximum distress. As was continually pointed out, child ill-health was economically disastrous, with a key element of the nation's 'capital' being wasted. At a time when the whole of the Western world seemed on the verge of collapse, this concern with the future, in the form of the nation's children, was understandable. The situation was exacerbated by serious doubts over the shortcomings of existing services. The school meals service, for example, had been set up partly at Labour instigation, but even by 1939 was extremely limited in scope. Inadequacies were also evident in school medical service statistics, thereby throwing doubt on the efficacy of the service itself. The increased emphasis on nutrition heightened such concerns.[31]

This stress on nutrition was related to the increasingly 'scientific' nature of medicine. In a significant conflation of two of the sections of the Labour Party most concerned with child welfare, the SJCIWO set up a sub-committee on child nutrition in 1932, onto which it invited two members of the SMA, Somerville Hastings and Alfred Salter. This committee, as far as Labour women were concerned, generated much useful publicity.[32] Labour doctors, and particularly those of the SMA, were indeed active in arguing the need for adequate child nutrition. A columnist in *The Socialist Doctor* in 1934 acknowledged that medical science remained inexact, but suggested that malnutrition and undernutrition must 'be of commoner occurrence than is generally acknowledged'. Hence the need for the growth in, and greater dissemination of, information on nutrition.[33]

The 'scientific' approach propagated by socialist doctors influenced others in the Labour movement. Barbara Drake argued that in a 'civilised community' children had the 'first claim' on the nation's food resources. This had been acknowledged in wartime but now, when the supply and variety of foodstuffs were greater than before, many children were 'living on diets which do not even provide the minimum conditions of health and growth'. Drake also refuted suggestions that school feeding would undermine parental responsibility, a long-standing Conservative jibe, and further concluded that with more widespread school feeding a start would be made on planning both the allocation of national food resources and children's diets. This would ultimately lead to the improvement of the nation's health and physique.[34] There were many other examples of such arguments, some sophisticated and consciously 'scientific'. Others were more ambiguous and provocative, for example the pieces in *The Labour Woman* entitled 'Malnutrition – The Government's Policy', and 'The Starvation of the People'.[35] One important recurring theme in this literature was the belief that, as Susan Lawrence put it, 'If we are getting a C.3 population, this fact can be measured', although virtually all Labour commentators were highly sceptical of official statistics – as a report of 1936 put it, the 'value of official statistics relating to the nutrition of school children must be questioned'. Nonetheless the prominent Labour peer Lord Snell, a former MP and LCC chairman, could claim at the BMA nutrition conference that 'the existence of chronic under-feeding was well-established and need not be argued at any length'. Snell went on to draw on his LCC experience, concluding that some educational expenditure was wasted because of the 'ill-nourished condition of some of the children'.[36]

What 'scientific' evidence confirmed for Labour was what observation and experience had always suggested: that malnourishment was part of working-class child life, associated as it was with poverty and, especially in the 1930s, unemployment. This scientism, in itself almost certainly related to the contemporary obsession with 'planning', also appeared to provide a rational basis for future progress and for countering the National Government's complacency. As Somerville Hastings put it, if 'we are to put up a strong and effective case' against reductions in the standard of living, 'we must know exactly what are our human needs'.[37] Children were therefore objects of concern not simply in their own right. As never before they represented the future. This appeared threatened by physical and mental deterioration. Consequently, any economic recovery and any advance towards socialism would be extremely hard to come by. Scientism also clearly influenced the Labour movement debate on family allowances, in that one important element in the argument against cash allowances was the alleged inability of the working-class mother to fully understand the proper nutritional requirements of her children.

CONCLUSION

The concern within the Labour Party, and indeed the wider Labour movement, over child welfare in the inter-war period was largely conditioned by the pressures of domestic and international politics and the claims of malnutrition and of nutritional science. There was, consequently, a perceived need to clarify the aims, philosophy and organisation of the child welfare services.

What was the historical significance of this concern? Did the Labour Party have, by 1939, a clear view of its child welfare policies and the sort of services and structures these would involve? The answers to these questions are not straightforward. On the one hand, Labour had rejected cash family allowances in favour of collective services such as school meals and a child health service. The party was prepared to mount national campaigns on, for example, the provision of milk to the under-5s, an important nutritional issue.[38] At local level Labour representatives were able to make improvements in child welfare facilities, with the LCC frequently cited as an example of what could be achieved. And, as Graves and Thane both point out, local child welfare work was often carried out by women, once again emphasising the significance of both localism and gender in Labour's welfare activities.[39]

On the other hand, it would be wrong to suggest that official Labour policy constituted a coherent and comprehensive child welfare programme, or that it had fully addressed the organising and financing of such policies. Not least was this because of the relationship between the leadership and bodies such as the women's organisations and the SMA. Labour was clearly anxious in the inter-war years to win over newly enfranchised women, and women's organisations such as the SJCIWO and the Women's

Co-operative Guild were central in pressing child welfare issues. In Labour local authorities women were instrumental in improving welfare conditions for children. But their status within the party as a whole was more ambiguous and problematical. The SJCIWO was able to get the *Children's Charter* published by the Labour Party. But this did not mean that the party necessarily endorsed it; indeed the rubric to the pamphlet made it clear that it was the outcome of a report initiated and discussed by Labour women, and not by the party as a whole. The official Labour Party could therefore use such publications as propaganda while remaining uncommitted to their detail. This in turn highlights gender relations within the Party as a whole, although it is also noticeable that women among the leadership were usually prepared to follow the leadership line.[40]

With the Socialist Medical Association a similar story, if for different reasons, presented itself. The Labour Party was clearly glad to receive 'expert' advice on matters such as nutrition, when medicine was taking on a much more 'scientific' bent. But as with the *Children's Charter*, it was significant that the Party leadership was careful not to give official sanction to key SMA documents, despite these containing, *inter alia*, wide-ranging child welfare proposals. The problem here was that while female and medical bodies were seen as having important propaganda functions, they were not allowed to dictate the pace of Party policy. Thus while Hastings' evidence to the family allowances committee might have been useful in sanctioning already-existing ideas, his more radical demands for comprehensive child welfare provision were much more problematical. This in turn points to the inherent caution of the Labour leadership, especially over finance.[41]

Senior Labour politicians were unspecific in their proposals for welfare, including child welfare, provision. 'Planning', a vogue word of the 1930s, was usually assumed to mean economic rather than social planning. The economy, it was felt, had to be sorted out prior to any real consideration of the nature and shape of welfare services, and consequently social policy proposals were for the most part ill-defined or simply propagandistic. Added to this was the as yet unresolved problem of how to create comprehensive welfare provision from the existing patchwork of local, voluntarist and state services. This resulted in a situation not quantitatively or qualitatively much further on from the notoriously vague proposals of 1918. As Marwick points out, the 'unproductiveness of Labour's social thought in the 1930s' is striking. Power relationships within the party continued to exclude bodies such as Labour women or the SMA from having a decisive say in formulating policy, with leadership caution tending to triumph over female or medical radicalism.[42]

The inter-war Labour Party at all levels was committed to improving the condition of Britain's children. It identified itself as the party of childhood, and was proud of its past achievements. This concern with child welfare derived from a number of sources. Gender was important, child-related policies being seen as particularly appealing to newly enfranchised female voters. Similarly, many Labour women were active in both providing local child welfare services, and in agitating for such services. Indeed it is noticeable how much of the discussion on child welfare took place in the women's organisations and in the journal *The Labour Woman*. At a deeper and more complex level, it is also the case that much of the political and electoral propaganda on child welfare made implicit or explicit assumptions about the traditional family role for women. This in turn is a significant comment on both male and female Labour Party attitudes. An analysis of Labour propaganda representations of women and children – including in such journals as *The Labour Woman* – would be deeply revealing. The failure of the Labour Party as a whole to adopt a coherent national programme on child welfare was an indicator of gender relationships within the Party. In the last resort, economic and industrial matters took priority at the expense of social welfare proposals, a reflection of the weight of organised male trade unionism in Labour power structures.

Other factors apart from gender had a role to play in structuring Labour Party concern over child welfare. Children were seen as the future saviours of democracy in a world where, by the 1930s, democracy was under considerable attack. They were therefore not just an economic 'investment', but also a political 'investment'. The findings of nutritional science and the onset of deep economic depression made such concerns all the more urgent. This diversity of factors influencing attitudes to child welfare might be seen as evidence of Pedersen's point that, on occasions, overemphasis on gender can obscure the fact that 'many social policies are concerned less with men or women than with children; gender relations are not always the central concern'.[43] Once again, however, the question needs to be posed: given

Labour's concern for children, for whatever reasons, why was it that no clear and coherent programme of child welfare had emerged by 1939?

The answer to this in large part is indicative of the more general lack of clarity in the Party's thinking on social welfare. Fiscal responsibility and the emphasis on economic planning resulted in an inability to see child welfare, or any other form of welfare, in anything other than the most general, rhetorical, terms. Labour was undoubtedly committed to improving the lot of the nation's children, but beyond tinkering with already existing mechanisms and institutions had no clear idea of how to do this. The idea of 'investing' in children for the sake of the future had immense emotional and political appeal, but how this was to be funded was much more problematical. It was only with the coming of World War II and Labour's adoption of the tools of Keynesian economic management and the structures of Beveridge's proposals that solutions appeared to be on offer. Labour's inter-war concern with child welfare is therefore significant in itself in showing how concerns over the state of the nation and the future of democracy came to be focused on children. But it also illustrates the limitations of Labour thinking on welfare and, more generally, the complex interaction of political, economic, social and intellectual factors which go into health and welfare policy formation.

NOTES

1 I am grateful to Anne Digby, Harry Hendrick, John Macnicol and Charles Webster for their comments on this chapter.
2 The Labour Party, *Children First! Labour's Policy Described*, London, The Labour Party, 1929, p. 3; The Labour Party, *A Children's Charter*, London, The Labour Party, 1937; *Report of the Thirty Seventh Annual Conference of the Labour Party*, London, The Labour Party, 1937, p. 24.
3 G. D. H. Cole, 'Health in the Schools', *New Statesman*, 22 November 1924, p. 195.
4 John Stewart, 'J. R. MacDonald, the Labour Party and Child Welfare, 1900–1914', *Twentieth Century British History*, vol. 4, no. 2, 1993.
5 Philip Snowden, *Labour and the New World*, London, The Labour Party, 1921, pp. 13, 236 – see also his *If Labour Rules*, London, The Labour Party, 1923, p. 42; Draft Report of a Special Committee Appointed by the Labour Party, *Motherhood and Child Endowment*, London, The Labour Party, 1921, p. 19; Mary Sutherland, 'A Children's Charter', *The Labour Woman*, July 1937, pp. 104–5; *Report*

of the Thirty First Annual Conference of the Labour Party, London, The Labour Party, pp. 66–7.

6 Draft Report of a Special Committee, *Motherhood*, p. 4.

7 David Jarvis, 'Mrs. Maggs and Betty: The Conservative Appeal to Women Voters in the 1920s', *Twentieth Century British History*, vol. 5, no. 2, 1994.

8 *Cooperative Representatives in Parliament*, Manchester, The Labour Party, 1924, p. 23; The Labour Party, *Women and the General Election*, London, The Labour Party, 1929, p. 28, also quoted in *The Labour Woman*, February 1929, p. 23. That the leadership were highly sensitive to the question of women's votes can be seen, for example, in their concerns over a by-election defeat in Ilford in September 1920, which was attributed to the majority of women voting against Labour. A report on this can be found in the National Executive Committee (NEC) files. For the impact of the female franchise, and further examples of Labour propaganda directed at women, see Jorgen Rasmussen, 'Women in Labour: The Flapper Vote and Party System Transformation in Britain', *Electoral Studies*, 1984, vol. 3.

9 Barbara Ayrton Gould, 'The Nursery School Child', *The Labour Woman*, December 1932, p. 185.

10 *Minutes of the Executive Committee of the Labour Party*, 8 February 1927.

11 *The Labour Woman*, October 1930, p. 152; Averil D. Sanderson Furniss, 'The Citizenship of Women', in Herbert Tracey (ed.), *The Book of the Labour Party, Vol. 2*, London, The Labour Party, 1925, pp. 255ff; *Report of the Twenty Third Annual Conference of the Labour Party*, London, The Labour Party, 1923, p. 247; TUC and the Labour Party, *Joint Committee on the Living Wage etc; Interim Report on Family Allowances and Child Welfare*, London, TUC/Labour Party, 1928, pp. 30, 17–18; Hilary Land, 'The Introduction of Family Allowances', in Phoebe Hall, Hilary Land, Roy Parker and Adrian Webb (eds), *Change, Choice and Conflict in Social Policy*, London, Heinemann, 1975, pp. 166ff; Pat Thane, 'Women of the British Labour Party and Feminism', in H. L. Smith (ed.), *British Feminism in the Twentieth Century*, Aldershot, Edward Elgar, 1990, p. 139; Idem, 'Visions of Gender in the Making of the British Welfare State', in Gisella Bock and Pat Thane (eds), *Maternity and Gender Policies*, London, Routledge, 1991, pp. 107ff; Hilary Land, 'Eleanor Rathbone and the Economy of the Family', in Smith (ed.), *British Feminism*, p. 117; Susan Pedersen, *Family, Dependence, and the Origins of the Welfare State*, Cambridge, Cambridge University Press, 1993, p. 166. For the argument that Labour policy increasingly came to deny the claims for economic independence by women, see Caroline Rowan, 'Women in the Labour Party', *Feminist Review*, 1982, vol. 12, pp. 79ff.

12 *Minutes of the Executive Committee of the Labour Party*, 26 and 27 March 1930. An attempt by Arthur Henderson to re-open the issue, despite TUC resistance, came to nothing: *Minutes of the Executive Committee of the Labour Party*, 28 and 29 January 1931; John Macnicol, *The Movement for Family Allowances*, London,

Heinemann, 1980, pp. 144ff; Pedersen, *Family*, pp. 197ff; TUC General Council, *Family Allowances: Text of the Minority and Majority Reports issued by the TUC and Labour Party Joint Committee – Verbatim Report of the Debate at the Nottingham Congress*, London, TUC, 1930. The vote on the General Council, taken on 28 May 1930, in favour of the Minority Report was 16 to 8: see the memorandum prepared for the Economic Committee of the TUC, *TUC Economic Committee: Family Allowances*, 7 March 1939. The Labour Party debated the issue at the 1930 conference: *Report of the Thirtieth Annual Conference of the Labour Party*, London, The Labour Party, 1930, pp. 174ff.

13 TUC, *Family Allowances*, pp. 4–5; TUC and the Labour Party, *Joint Committee*, pp. 31, 27, 23; *The Labour Woman*, August 1930, pp. 121–2. For a fuller discussion of Hastings' approach to child welfare, see John Stewart, 'Socialist Proposals for Health Reform in Inter-War Britain: The Case of Somerville Hastings', *Medical History*, July 1995.

14 Frances Edwards, in *The Labour Woman*, September 1930, p. 137. Hastings replied to such critics, arguing, rather disingenuously, that he was not against family allowances *per se*, but rather that the available resources could be better employed. He again stressed that with the best will in the world mothers did not *necessarily* know what was best for their children – *The Labour Woman*, October 1930, p. 153. But to suggest, as does Graves, that Hastings objected to cash payments solely on the basis of the alleged ineptitude of working-class mothers is only a partial analysis of the case: Pamela Graves, *Labour Women*, Cambridge, Cambridge University Press, 1994, p. 107.

15 John Macnicol, 'Welfare, Wages and the Family: Child Endowment in Comparative Perspective, 1900–1950', in Roger Cooter (ed.), *In the Name of the Child*, London, Routledge, 1992. I am grateful to John Macnicol for his comments on Labour's attitude to cash benefits of the family allowance type.

16 TUC, *Family Allowances*, p. 14; British Medical Association, *Nutrition and the Public Health: Proceedings of a National Conference on the Wider Aspects of Nutrition, April 27th–29th, 1939*, London, BMA, 1940, pp. 112ff.

17 The Labour Party, *A Children's Charter*, pp. 2–3.

18 Pedersen, *Family*, p. 199; Pat Thane, 'Women in the British Labour Party and the Construction of State Welfare, 1906–1939', in Seth Koven and Sonya Michel (eds), *Mothers of a New World*, London, Routledge, 1993.

19 John Stevenson and Chris Cook, *The Slump*, London, Quartet, 1977, p. 277 see local politics, particularly those of effective social reform, as important in Labour's survival; Beatrice Webb, 'The End of the Poor Law', in Marion Phillips (ed.), *Women and the Labour Party*, London, Headley Bros, 1918, p. 50 – this also contains important essays on child welfare by Margaret Llewelyn Davies and Margaret McMillan; *The Labour Woman*, October 1925, p. 169; A. Susan

186   John Stewart

Lawrence, 'Labour's Road to Public Health', *The Labour Woman*,
October 1929, p. 152. The American political scientist McHenry noted
the increased expenditure on child health and welfare in Labour-
controlled areas, although he was sceptical about the lack of a nationally defined municipal programme: Dean McHenry, *The Labour Party
in Transition*, London, George Routledge, 1938, pp. 202ff.

20 The Labour Party, *Preserve the Real Wealth of the Nation* (leaflet no.
203), London, The Labour Party, 1928. James Maxton of the ILP did
accuse the government of child murder, but this was exceptional:
Charles Loch Mowat, *Britain between the Wars*, London, Methuen,
1968, p. 155; *Report of Twenty Second Annual Conference of the
Labour Party*, London, The Labour Party, 1922, p. 230.

21 Fenner Brockway, *Bermondsey Story: The Life of Alfred Salter*,
London, Allen & Unwin, 1949, pp. 101–2; H. R. S. Phillpott, *Where
Labour Rules*, London, Methuen, 1934, pp. 70ff, 41ff; The Labour
Party, *Local Government Speaker's Handbook*, London, The Labour
Party, 1937–8 edn, pp. 10–24; The Labour Party, *Vote Labour and
Give Us a Chance* (leaflet no. 78), London, The Labour Party, 1938;
Socialist Medical Association Records, Brynmor Jones Library,
University of Hull, file DSM (2) 5, Miscellaneous Correspondence.

22 See, for example, *London County Council Annual Report 1937*,
London, LCC, 1938, vol. III (part II), Report for the year 1937 of
the School Medical Officer; Malcolm Richardson, 'Education and
Politics between the Wars', in Andrew Saint (ed.), *The Politics and
People of London*, London, Hambledon Press, 1989; and, on the
limited nature of LCC reforms, G. D. H. Cole (ed.), *A Short History
of the British Working Class Movement, 1789–1947*, London, Allen &
Unwin, 1947, p. 442.

23 The Labour Party, *Your Britain*, London, The Labour Party, 1937,
p. 6; Katharine Bruce Glasier, 'Victory for Socialism – The First
Twelve Months', *The Labour Woman*, May 1935, p. 73.

24 Mary Sutherland, 'The Right to Health', *The Labour Woman*, July
1936, p. 104; see, as an example of the left's criticisms of the phys-
ical education campaign, most editions of the Socialist Medical
Association's journal, *Medicine Today and Tomorrow* and the 'Health
and Nutrition' file of the Labour Party Research Department, Labour
Party archives, Manchester; Lucy Noel-Buxton, 'The Nation's Health',
The Labour Woman, May 1937, p. 72; John Welshman, *The School
Medical Service in England and Wales, 1907–1939*, University of
Oxford, DPhil. thesis, 1988, pp. 237–44.

25 *Parliamentary Debates*, 5th Series, 1935–6, vol. 314, col. 1230; *Report
of the Thirty Sixth Annual Conference of the Labour Party*, London,
The Labour Party, 1936, p. 42.

26 *Parliamentary Debates*, 5th Series, 1935–6, vol. 314, col. 1266.

27 Hugh Dalton, *Practical Socialism for Britain*, London, George
Routledge, 1935, p. 324.

28 *The Labour Woman*, September 1922, pp. 141, 146; *Report of the
Nineteenth Annual Conference of the Labour Party*, London, The
Labour Party, 1919, p. 164.

29 TUC General Council and Labour Party Executive Committee: Joint Research and Information Department, Advisory Committee on Public Health, *Notes on the Effect of Unemployment on the Health of Children*, memo no. 41, May 1922.

30 The Labour Party, *The Health of the Nation: Why Are We C.3?* (leaflet no. 217), London, The Labour Party, 1929; The Labour Party, *Children First!*, p. 10; The Labour Party, *Appalling Health Record of 'National' Government*, London, The Labour Party, 1935.

31 Among the many non-Labour approaches to this issue are: C. E. McNally, *Public Ill Health*, London, Gollancz, 1935, ch. V; and Marjorie Green, *Malnutrition Among School Children*, Children's Minimum Council, 1938; on the limitations of the school meals service see Charles Webster, 'The Health of the School Child During the Depression', in N. Parry and D. McNair (eds), *The Fitness of the Nation*, Leicester, History of Education Society, 1983, passim; and Welshman, *School Medical*, ch. 4, and especially pp. 167, 175.

32 *Minutes of the General Purposes Committee of the Standing Joint Committee of Industrial Women's Organisations*, 8 December 1932; *Minutes of the Standing Joint Committee of Industrial Women's Organisations*, 9 March 1933.

33 'Caractacus', 'How Are the Children? The Assessment of Malnutrition', *The Socialist Doctor*, vol. 2, no. 3, 1934, pp. 11–12.

34 Barbara Drake, *Starvation in the Midst of Plenty: A New Plan for the State Feeding of School Children*, London, The Fabian Society, 1933, pp. 4, 15–16; Barbara Drake, *Nutrition: A Policy of National Health*, London, New Fabian Research Bureau, 1936, pp. 23–4, 35–6. In her 'Introduction' to this last work, Eleanor Rathbone argued that it was 'considerations ... fundamentally military' which had forced malnutrition into the foreground of public affairs.

35 'Malnutrition – The Government's Policy', *The Labour Woman*, June 1935, p. 93; Susan Lawrence, 'The Starvation of the People', *The Labour Woman*, May 1933, p. 74.

36 Susan Lawrence, 'Are We Underfed?', *The Labour Woman*, October 1935, p. 153; The Labour Party, *Reports on Nutrition and Food Supplies and Women in Offices*, London, The Labour Party, 1936, p. 5; BMA, *Nutrition*, p. 91. On the debates over the accuracy of nutrition statistics, see Welshman, *School Medical*, pp. 148ff. For the general context, see Harry Hendrick, *Child Welfare in England*, London, Routledge, 1994, pp. 136ff.

37 For planning see Arthur Marwick, 'Middle Opinion in the Thirties: Planning, Progress and Political "Agreement"', *English Historical Review*, vol. LXXIX, April 1964. Somerville Hastings, *A National Physiological Minimum*, London, The Fabian Society, p. 3.

38 See, for example, the TUC General Council: Education Committee, *Draft of Evidence to be Given to the Board of Education Consultative Committee on Infant and Nursery Schools*, 19 September 1932, p. 3; The Labour Party, *Socialism and the Condition of the People*, London, The Labour Party, 1934, p. 17. For details of the debates over milk provision, see Welshman, *School Medical*, pp. 158–62, 185–8.

39 Graves, *Labour*, ch. 5; Thane, 'Visions of Gender', p. 106.

40 The Labour Party, *A Children's Charter*, p. 1. On the relationship of women to the Labour Party see Martin Pugh, *Women and the Women's Movement in Britain, 1914–1959*, London, Macmillan, 1992, pp. 129ff; and Brian Harrison, *Prudent Revolutionaries*, Oxford, Oxford University Press, 1987, pp. 125ff.

41 Stewart, 'Socialist Proposals'; on the Labour Party and fiscal caution see, for example, K. J. Hancock, 'The Reduction of Unemployment as a Problem of Public Policy', *English Historical Review*, 1962–3, vol. 15.

42 For the immediate post-war era, see The Labour Party, *Labour and the New Social Order*, London, The Labour Party, 1918, p. 5; see also, for example, the vague and unspecific proposals in Arthur Greenwood, *Immediate Steps Towards the New Social Order*, London, The Labour Party, 1933, passim, and The Labour Party, *General Election 1935: The Labour Party's Call to Power*, London, The Labour Party, 1935, p. 2. Arthur Marwick, 'The Labour Party and the Welfare State in Britain, 1900–1948', *American Historical Review*, December 1967, p. 395. For the general context, see David Howell, *British Social Democracy*, London, Croom Helm, 1976, chs 2 and 3, where he points out the ambiguities at the heart of Labour proposals by the late 1930s; Richard Lyman, 'The British Labour Party: the Conflict between Socialist Ideas and Practical Politics between the Wars', *Journal of British Studies, 1965*, vol. v, no. 1, where he points to the break between pre- and post-World War II attitudes; and Paul Addison, *The Road to 1945*, London, Pimlico, rev. edn. 1994, ch. 1, where he points out Labour's caution and relative vagueness of social reform aims. José Harris argues the continuing antipathy to the state, including among those on the political left: 'Political Ideas and the Debate on State Welfare, 1940–45', in H. L. Smith (ed.), *War and Social Change*, Manchester, Manchester University Press, 1986, p. 236. For a rather more 'optimistic' view of the Labour Party in the inter-war period, see Charles Webster, 'The Labour Party and the Origins of the National Health Service', in Nicolaas Rupke (ed.), *Science, Politics and the Public Good*, London, Macmillan, 1988, p. 198, although this in turn might be qualified by his 'Health, Welfare and Unemployment During the Depression', *Past and Present*, 1985, vol. 109, p. 229. Similarly, the opening remarks in Ray Earwicker, 'The Emergence of a Medical Strategy in the Labour Movement, 1906–1919', *Bulletin of the Society for the Social History of Medicine*, 1981, vol. 29, are pertinent here.

43 Pedersen, *Family*, p. 11.

Chapter 8

Gender, welfare and old age in Britain, 1870s–1940s

Pat Thane

This essay explores some of the ways in which gender can, and cannot, be used as a tool for analysing the history of social welfare in Britain by focusing upon the experiences of older people. Men and women can experience different types of need and may experience need differently. Different types of policy may evolve in response to their differing experiences. They may play different roles in policy making and have different policy objectives. '*May*' in all these cases, not 'must,' since clearly the differences between the life experiences of the sexes are not absolute and gender is not the only characteristic that divides people. Nevertheless gender is an important category of analysis which still has not been sufficiently integrated into studies of the history of British social welfare.

For as long as systematic demographic records have been available in Britain (since registration of births, marriages and deaths became compulsory in the 1840s), and indeed for much longer, more women than men have lived past their mid-60s – the age long conventionally if arbitrarily applied as the boundary between 'middle age' and 'old age'. Old women are more likely to be poor than old men, due to their lesser lifetime opportunities to accumulate resources. Because of these differences and also the different work experiences of women and men, different policy remedies have been suggested and implemented in relation to their needs. Also, women and men have often stood in different relationships to policy-making for the elderly and to the administration of such measures as emerged. This has not been a simple matter of male inclusion and female exclusion in the policy-making and administrative processes.

This becomes especially obvious if we shift the focus of discussion from the central state to take account of local government and the voluntary sector, which has always been large in Britain. Even in the nineteenth century women were not wholly excluded from the public, policy-making and administrative sphere, though their role was more limited than that of men. Women could be elected to local government office, and female householders had the local vote from 1869, although none of them could vote at national level or enter Parliament until 1918.[1] Also, women in the nineteenth and twentieth centuries were prominent in voluntary organisations and pressure groups, often playing leadership roles and initiating policy as well as acting as unpaid social workers.[2]

THE WELFARE OF THE ELDERLY POOR IN PRE-INDUSTRIAL ENGLAND

It was only towards the end of the nineteenth century in Britain that old age *as such* came to be defined in popular and political discourse as a social problem. This was not because old people were for the first time surviving in significant numbers. People over 60 formed 9 per cent of the total population of England through the second half of the seventeenth century, and between 8 and 9 per cent through the eighteenth century. They made up a lower percentage of total population (under 7) for most of the nineteenth century, due mainly to the high birth rate.[3] Victorian Britain was an unusually young society. It should be remembered that the age structure of any society is more likely to be determined by birth rates than by death rates, except in periods of unusually sharp fluctuations in mortality. The proportion of old people in the population rose slightly at the end of the nineteenth century, though it remained below eighteenth-century levels. Thereafter it climbed steadily due to the combined effects of a falling birth rate and declining adult death rates (see Table 8.1).

Nor was it the case that the poverty, ill-health and other needs of many old people were previously unrecognised or unprovided for by services financed either from taxation or by voluntary contributions. A statutory poor law, funded from local taxation, had existed in England and Wales from the late sixteenth century (Scotland had a different history) and it is increasingly clear that this had its antecedents in regular local initiatives from at least the fourteenth century onwards by towns and villages to levy local funds to assist their local poor.[4]

Table 8.1 Percentage of population aged 65 and over, Great Britain, 1851–1981

Census year	%	Census year	%
1851	4.6	1951	10.9
1881	4.6	1971	13.2
1911	5.2	1981	15.1
1931	7.4		

Source: P. Thane, 'Old Age: Burden or Benefit', in H. Joshi (ed.), *The Changing Population of Britain*, Oxford, Blackwell, 1989, p. 57.

It is important for understanding later policy developments to recognise that in England there was a commitment from a very early date on the part of the *community* to provide for the poor, or at least those who were respectable,very poor and settled local residents. Strangers or the disreputable were much less certain of provision. The collectivity assisted those of the elderly poor who could not provide for themselves by work or otherwise, who had no surviving adult children or whose children were themselves too poor to give more than minimal support to failing parents. It was assumed that where children survived, if they had not migrated far away and possessed the necessary resources, they would do what they could to provide emotional and material support for their elderly parents. But it was recognised that, given high mortality rates, parents often outlived their children. It has been estimated that in the later middle ages between 20 and 30 per cent of men and women had no living child at their deaths; survival rates remained similar until the nineteenth century. Infant and adult mortality rates remained high through the sixteenth, seventeenth and eighteenth centuries; and between 10 and 20 per cent of marriages were childless. Also from medieval times English society was geographically highly mobile. With the early dwindling of a peasantry rooted in the land and expanding international links this mobility increased over the centuries, sometimes severing ties between the generations. Even when the children of poor old people survived and lived nearby, on good terms with their parents, they were often poor themselves. Indeed, elderly parents were all too likely to become dependent at a point at which their offspring's children were at peak dependency.

For all of these reasons old people often could not be supported by their children. It was certainly not the norm or the expectation that old people would live with their children. Over the centuries, elderly people seem to have sought to remain for as long as possible in their accustomed homes, often supported by an un- married child, sometimes moving in with a married son or daughter for a short time before death, but if forced to leave their accustomed homes at least as likely to lodge with strangers as with kin. This does not imply that they necessarily severed emotional or material ties with their children, but most people displayed a clear preference for retaining as much independence as possible until as late an age as possible.[5] The fact that old people lived alone should not, then as now, be interpreted to mean that they were necessarily isolated and neglected. The generations could be mutually supportive even when they did not live together. Nor were older men or women necessarily helpless and dependent. The flow of provision could be from older to younger as well as *vice versa*. Old people could be decisive agents of their own fates.[6]

The statutory poor law from 1601 did state that children should be responsible for the needs of elderly parents, but in practice this was often disregarded by administrators of the law, due to the absence or poverty of the children. Rather the community acknowledged a responsibility (paid for from local taxation or local charitable donations) to provide such support as old people could not acquire through self-help – in particular, engaging in paid work until as late an age as possible – or from kin and neigh- bours. Old people were the most frequent recipients of poor relief. In most times and places old women and younger widowed mothers made greater use of poor relief than did men, due to their more restricted access to adequately-paid work and other resources. Poverty has long been feminine.

The poor law could play such an active role partly because England was, in comparison with other countries of northern Europe, for example Scotland, long relatively prosperous; income and wealth were widely enough spread for such transfers to be possible. This of course does not explain why such practices became the norm. Societies do not necessarily help the poor merely because they can afford it. In part it was a form of insurance, since even moderately prosperous landholders might fall, childless, onto hard times with advancing age; nor was the

presence of impoverished, starving, begging old people a contribution to social order. To provide minimally for the poor was one
of the means to maintain order in the community. Such measures
emerged out of communal self-interest and communal pressure.
The processes by which the decisions were reached at at local
level, where the national poor law was interpreted and administered, cannot easily be reconstructed but it is probable that the
women of the local community, the traditional keepers and
promoters of local custom in respect of social relations, played a
part. Parish relief was complemented by voluntary charity of
amounts which varied from place to place.

The resulting provision was hardly lavish for elderly people,
whose earlier lives would normally have been lived at a low
standard of subsistence. But relief under the old poor law, before
it was revised in 1834, was not always punitive or stigmatising and
it was wide-ranging in the services it provided, though there was
considerable variation in practice among different places and over
time. Old people might be provided with medicine, nursing care
(often by other older women paid by the parish), accommodation, either in almshouses or in the homes of others, often of poor
widows; or old men and women were given paid work about the
parish or assisted to continue in their accustomed trades. Women,
sometimes themselves old, had an important role as providers of
care for the more dependent old people and older women seem
sometimes to have been more valued and honoured than old men
by reason of their knowledge of, for example, herbal medicine.
The stereotype of the solitary, poor old woman, marginalised from
the community and vulnerable to accusations of witchcraft, has
not stood up to recent scrutiny. The useful, respected older
woman, sharing her home with others equally or more needy, is
closer to reality.

Some historians have gone so far as to describe this system of
the sixteenth to early nineteenth centuries as 'a welfare state in
miniature'.[7] There were, however, important respects in which this
old poor law differed from the twentieth-century welfare state.
One was in its central emphasis upon the importance of work
and self-help. Poor relief was emphatically only a supplement
available when an individual, with all due effort,was unable to
support himself or, more often, herself. Another difference was
that no one had a statutory right to any form of relief; all relief
was a matter of local discretion, though according to custom it

became normal for respectable old people or widows to receive the help they needed.

Also, no one received poor relief simply because he or she was old and there was no fixed age at which payments became due to old people. Old and otherwise 'impotent' people without other resources might become regular 'poor law pensioners', as historians have called them, receiving regular amounts of weekly relief. They received it because they were incapable of supporting themselves ('impotent') and destitute rather than because they were old, and payment could begin at any age from 50 to 80 or more, or at much younger ages for the seriously disabled. Need, and indeed old age itself, was defined by physical capacity rather than by chronological age. In poor law records of the eighteenth century one woman was regularly described as 'old' when in her fifties. Another who died in her seventies was never so described.[8] There was a widely acknowledged individual variability in the experience of ageing. The social problem for which relief was provided was defined as destitution and incapacity for self-help, not old age itself.

THE DEMAND FOR OLD AGE PENSIONS

Only in the later nineteenth century was old age *as such* defined as a social problem; a predictable cause of need, with a more or less predictable chronological starting point, requiring remedy from the communal purse. This was when the demand began for a state old age pension. What the pensionable age should be varied among proponents, from 55 upwards though it was most often 60 or 65. However, working-class representatives especially argued that no single age was suitable because individuals deteriorated at such variable ages.

The campaign for a state old age pension was active from the late 1870s. In 1908 a pension of 5 shillings per week (25p) was introduced, payable at age 70 to those with incomes below a fixed amount and subject to certain other conditions.[9] The campaign followed a significant diminution in the flexibility and relative generosity of the poor law. On a national level this began in 1834 when the law was amended to make poor relief more restrictive and stigmatising. It most severely affected old people, and also widows and separated wives, in the 1870s when there was a national attempt to abolish relief payments to people in their own homes and to force them to choose between the workhouse and independence. Old people and widows had continued to be the most regular recipients of 'outdoor relief', as it was called. At the same time sons and daughters were put under stronger pressure than before to support their elderly parents. They could be, and were, prosecuted in larger numbers than before for repayment of any relief paid to their parents.[10]

The thinking behind the change of policy appears to have been that England (Scottish poor law practice was still different) had become a much wealthier society in which, unlike in any past time, individuals could reasonably be expected to be self-helping. Increasingly, it was argued, trade unions and friendly societies provided pensions for their members or old people could purchase annuities at the state-owned Post Office. Alternatively, it was believed their children could better afford to care for them than in the past. Failing that, it was thought that charity had grown to such proportions that it could effectively substitute for outdoor poor relief for the small numbers of respectable elderly or widowed poor.

All of these expectations proved erroneous. Few people of the stratum likely to be reduced to poor relief had enough surplus income to invest in annuities or even to pay the regular subscription to a friendly society or trade union; unions in any case were restricted to a small élite of workers and both very rarely admitted women. The problem remained that the children of the very poor were all too likely to be themselves poor, dead or migrated. Philanthropy had indeed greatly expanded during the nineteenth century. By how much has not yet been quantified, and perhaps cannot be, but the indications are that old people benefited less from this than other needy groups. In a youthful society there was more concern with children. Also the panic at the end of the century about the assumed physical deterioration of the population diverted charitable resources to the needs of mothers and infants and the health care of young people.

The chief outcome of the tightening up of the poor-relief system was an increase in numbers of old people in workhouses and increased reports of their starving in destitution rather than enter the workhouse. Hence the demands for a state pension to protect poor elderly people from this fate.

This background does not, however, explain the demand that it be paid at a fixed age. A possible alternative was a disability pension paid at whatever age regular work became impossible. In part the choice of a fixed pensionable age derived from the model of trade union, friendly society, and civil service pensions which were paid at fixed ages. Some large business firms were also beginning to introduce pensions at a fixed age, usually for their white-collar or highly-skilled staff. They saw it as a device to maintain a stable long-serving labour force and to enhance its efficiency by removing older workers who were assumed to be less efficient. The same argument had been made for introducing pensions at age 60 into the civil service in the 1850s. The fixed age eliminated the invidious problem for management of having to remove a worker at the point at which he or, much more rarely in pensionable occupations, she, became less capable.[11]

Such practices were still very unusual in British business at this time. It is notable that Britain reached the high level of industrialisation she was at by the end of the nineteenth century with a fixed retirement age still 'almost an unknown concept'.[12] However it was widely believed in the trade unions by the 1870s that employers were tending to ease workers out at earlier ages than before; also that older men who became unemployed were finding it harder to find re-employment. Hence the growth at this time of trade union superannuation schemes and workers' increasing support for a state pension for those who were not in unions.

According to the 1881 census, the first to contain information on retirement, more than 73 per cent of the male population of England and Wales aged over 65 was in paid employment. The percentage was 64.8 in 1891, 60.6 in 1901 and 56.0 in 1911. Eighteen per cent of women over 65 were recorded as being in paid employment in 1881, though female employment rates were regularly under-recorded in the nineteenth-century British census and have always to be used with caution.[13] The processes that lie behind these statistics are complex and not simply to be explained by changed management practices.[14] But certainly by the early years of the twentieth century some prominent employers were in favour of state pensions for the reasons of management given above. Given the characteristically small size of British firms, relatively few businesses felt able to provide their own pension schemes but preferred to pay through taxation for a state pension.

Hence part of the pressure for a state pension derived from concern at the plight of impoverished old men and women abandoned by the poor law. Another part, and in particular the demand for a fixed age defining the onset of old age, derived from changes that were, or were assumed to be, occurring mainly in the male sector of the gender-divided labour force. A prominent feature of the discourse around the demand for old age pensions was the description of pensions as the deserved reward of the male worker for long years of service to the national economy. However, the great majority of impoverished old people in this period were female. Only 37.5 per cent of the first state old age pensioners in 1909 were male (30.7 per cent in London); according to the 1911 census, 41.4 per cent of the over-70 population was male.

The two strands of the demand for pensions – as compensation for the greater stringency of the poor-relief system, or as compensation for enforced earlier retirement from the paid labour force – pointed towards different policy outcomes. The latter, which focused upon the needs of men, pointed towards an insurance pension financed by contributions from the beneficiary during working life; the former, which mainly provided for women, pointed towards wholly tax-financed pensions for beneficiaries who were too poor throughout their lives to make such contributions.

The initial demands were for insurance pensions. Trade unionists and other working people opposed this because they believed that most working-class people, especially women (as trade unionists pointed out), but also very many men in low-paid casual work, could not afford the weekly levy. Charles Booth, the social investigator, who knew more than most about the actual conditions of the aged poor, opposed the contributory principle on these grounds. He was the most prominent advocate of non-contributory old age pensions for all at 65, a proposal supported by the trade unions.[15] Insurance pensions were not appropriate for the very people who were most likely to experience severe poverty in old age.

By 1908, when the first state pensions scheme was drafted, it had become clear to the government and to the Treasury that the pressure for some form of pension had become too strong to be resisted, but that if it took a contributory form they would be faced with the costs of establishing an insurance scheme, with an outcry on behalf of the poorest who would be left out, and heavy expenditure on poor relief for this group for whom there was much public sympathy. They chose a non-contributory pension. The pensionable age was set as high as 70 and the pension was stringently means-tested in order to cut costs as far as possible. Nevertheless, more old people received the pension than had received poor relief; and an important new state benefit, the first cash benefit to be given outside the poor law, in practice mainly went to women.

Unlike the German insurance pensions introduced in 1889 (the first state pension in modern history[16]), but like the means-tested non-contributory schemes introduced in Denmark in 1891 and in New Zealand in 1898, the British system did not discriminate against women. The reasons for the differences lie in the different economic functions that pensions policies were expected to fulfil in the different countries. The German scheme was intended to induce skilled workers to support the political *status quo*. Elsewhere the priority was to deal with the problem that old people were gaining least from economic growth and that poor relief systems were inadequate mechanisms for ensuring that they did not slip unacceptably far behind other groups.

Britain introduced social insurance in 1911, covering most regularly employed manual workers, though not their partners or children, for health benefits and some of them also for periods of unemployment. The government refused to incorporate a disability pension into the health insurance scheme. These schemes did discriminate against women and casually employed men, relatively few of whom qualified; i.e. they provided for a different and to a great extent somewhat better-off sector of the working class than did the pension. Their purpose was less to relieve poverty than to maximise the work efficiency and sense of security of the more skilled workers by maintaining their health, and to discourage casual under-employment. National insurance was perceived as directly supportive of the needs of the economy and of political stability; old age pensions rather as a branch of the poor relief system. The outcome was a welfare system which reproduced the gender division of the work force. There were important differences of principle between them; insurance benefits were presented as a right of the contributor but pensions were not. At this stage of their development the difference was less stark: those receiving insurance benefits were policed and benefit could be withdrawn; whereas scrutiny of applicants for the pension appears to have been benign.

Another very important feature of the 1908 Pensions Act was that it constructed old age as beginning at a fixed age. It was an element in 'the socio-political structuring of the life course' which, as Christoph Conrad has pointed out, is an important consequence of state welfare practices.[17] It was a structuring modelled upon the male life cycle. Females more rarely than men, in the past as in the present, experienced retirement as an abrupt break in their lives; the important domestic roles which structure most women's lives, even if they are also in the paid labour force, continue. Age divisions as well as gender divisions shaped and were shaped by social policies.

THE INTRODUCTION OF INSURANCE PENSIONS AND THE LOWERING OF THE PENSION AGE FOR WOMEN

The pensionable age selected in Britain was higher than campaigners of all classes and both sexes had wanted. There was immediate pressure to reduce it to the preferred 65. This occurred in 1925 through the grafting of an insurance pension payable from age 65 onto the non-contributory scheme. Widows' and orphans' pensions were introduced at the same time. Thereafter, from 1928, all national insurance contributors received a pension at 65. Those who were not in insurable occupations continued to receive the non-contributory pension at 70. The two pensions were of the same amount. At its introduction, 10,445,000 men were in insurable employment and 4,645,000 women.[18] The first insurance pensions were paid in 1928 to 360,000 men and 177,000 women.[19] Only in 1946 did a married woman obtain a right to a pension by virtue of her husband's insurance, though of lower amount than a contributor's pension.

By 1925 the British government was more concerned than in 1908 to encourage a fixed and earlier retirement age for the employed labour force, partly in order to concentrate available work among younger workers at a time of high unemployment. This time it had other economic and political priorities than the relief of poverty in developing pensions policy. Being perceived as more marginal to the economy and to politics than men, old women were relatively disadvantaged.

There is little evidence of complaint from, or on behalf of, women at the exclusion of non-insured women from the extended pension scheme. However the grant of non-contributory widows' pensions in the same piece of legislation[20] to an undeniably needy group (they did not include war widows who were separately provided for), which women had long demanded, was seen as catering for the needs of the poorest women before as well as during old age.[21]

Once widows received pensions they normally retained them for life, so the problem of the lack of fit between the arbitrary pension age and biological age was removed for this particularly needy group of women. However, widows qualified initially only if they had care of children under the age of 14 at the time of their husband's death. This led to protest on behalf of older widows who got nothing until they qualified for the old age pension. It was argued, particularly by women's groups (and there were far more of them, far more active and articulate especially on social welfare issues in the 1920s and 1930s than much of the historiography would have it) who had campaigned for widows' pensions, that this was hard on women who had often long been out of the paid labour market, caring for husbands and children, and who would find difficulty in supporting themselves when widowed. In consequence the Labour government in 1929 introduced a pension equivalent to the old age pension for all widows aged 55 or above, as a transitional step towards paying them to all widows at the time of the death of the husband. After 1929 a significant number of women were receiving a permanent pension at earlier ages than men, as some compensation for their years of domestic labour and disadvantage in the labour market.

The pension was not an unconditional right. It was withdrawn if a widow remarried or cohabited. There is little sign that the cohabitation rule was oppressively policed. A total of 118 widows, out of many hundreds of thousands, lost their pensions for this reason in England and Wales between 1929 and 1939.[22] There were no complaints from a watchful women's movement. Surveillance was common to men and women under the national insurance system. Both could come under severe scrutiny if they were suspected of malingering while on sickness benefit; and the conditions on which unemployment insurance benefit could be obtained were stringent.

Some other women, especially unmarried women, came to resent the fact that widows received pensions at earlier ages than themselves. This was partly because they were conscious of another form of discrimination. Larger numbers of women were employed in insurable occupations by the 1930s and qualified for the pension at 65. White-collar employment had grown rapidly and become respectable for unmarried middle-class women. It was still unusual for a married middle-class woman to be in paid employment, indeed in many 'white blouse' occupations it was banned by the 'marriage bar'. Also, new forms of factory employment (e.g. in light engineering) were developing for working-class women. Larger numbers of 'spinsters', as they were described and called themselves – women who did not marry – spent their adult lives in permanent employment than had been the case before 1914. By the 1930s they were complaining that women found it hard to remain in employment until such a late age as men. Employers were said to be hostile to post-menopausal women and to ease them out of work before they qualified for their pension. Post-World War II surveys certainly did show considerable, irrational employer hostility to older women. Also it was argued that many middle-aged women gave up their jobs to care for elderly relatives, were unable to re-enter the labour market on the death of the relative and would not qualify for a pension until age 70, having fallen out of the insurance scheme.

In the 1930s there was an active campaign, led by the National Spinsters Association, for a lower state pension age for women, of 55 or 60. They argued that this would also benefit married couples. Since wives were on average five years younger than their husbands the lower age would enable them to retire simultaneously. They sought to draw upon still raw memories of the 'Great War', drawing an analogy between themselves and war widows, pointing out that the 'spinsterhood' of many of them was due to the deaths of so many men of their age. A government committee looked into the question in 1938–9. It found there was some, not overwhelming but real, evidence that women did lose their jobs at an earlier age than men, closer to 60 than 65; and the committee showed sympathy for the plight of those whom we would now call 'carers', who were left pensionless and often in considerable poverty after looking after their own elderly parents. It concluded that it was impossible to give pensions at an earlier age to 'spinsters' alongside widows, without provoking a furore from married women. Hence the Report recommended reducing the pensionable age to 60 for all women. This came about in 1940.

This success is hard to account for. The political force of the 'spinsters' was by no means irresistible. Perhaps the government was seeking to boost the morale of the female workforce who were so important to the war effort. The change certainly provided an opportunity to alter contribution rates in a manner that significantly increased the size of the insurance fund at a time when the government was seeking new sources of income to finance the war. In this, as in other aspects of pensions policy, a gender-centred analysis, though helpful, will not provide the whole explanation. (See also Chapter 3.)

INTERNATIONAL WOMEN'S CAMPAIGNS

Improved pension rights for women was the subject of international campaigns in the inter-war years which were linked with movements in individual countries. From the later nineteenth century there were extensive formal and informal contacts among women across the world concerning both women's and social welfare questions. International organisations were formed, such as the International Council of Women, and international congresses (in which women were prominent) were held on almost every conceivable aspect of social welfare. Such international contacts and organisations appear to have grown during the inter-war years. Women's organisations made the League of Nations a particular focus of their lobbying, and on questions of pensions and retirement its associated body, the International Labour Office, was the focus for pressure. It in turn encouraged member states to improve standards of employment and social security.

Significant numbers of women were appointed to the staff and to important committees of the League of Nations. Scandinavian and British women were especially active. It has been argued persuasively that they played an effective role in shifting the League and individual governments towards a more active commitment on issues of social welfare and women's rights.[23] Increasingly, if with limited success, women were using their new civil rights to promote and influence government policy.

THE BEVERIDGE REPORT AND AFTER

The British pensions and welfare systems were largely reconstructed after World War II; the social security system on the basis of the Beveridge Report of 1942. Beveridge had long been concerned to give recognition to the particular needs of women and to promote gender equality in the social security system. He was especially concerned that justice should be done to housewives who were not also in paid employment. He assumed, not unreasonably given past experience, that many women would continue in this role; he assumed that they *would*, rather than that they necessarily *should*. He proposed that they should acquire a right to a pension, though of a lesser amount than the husband's or a single working woman's, on the grounds that married women had fewer expenses, e.g. no rent to pay, this being the responsibility of the husband. Beveridge also proposed, however, that married women should be eligible for pensions not only in widowhood but on divorce or separation; and receive dependants' allowances during the husband's unemployment or sickness and an allowance for domestic help when sick themselves. While hardly fundamentally challenging conventional gender roles, he argued that the work of housewives was as important, socially and economically, as waged work and should be given equal recognition in the social security system. He described separation allowances as equivalent to allowances made to victims of industrial hazards.

Women's organisations at the time showed no great interest in the problems of deserted or divorced women, though they had done so previously. These proposals faced opposition from others on the grounds of 'subsidising sin'. They were reluctantly abandoned by Beveridge due to the difficulty of distinguishing 'innocent' from 'guilty' wives, thus leaving unsolved a set of problems which have since become more acute. The domestic benefit for sick housewives was dismissed by the Treasury on grounds of cost, as was Beveridge's attempt to include in the national insurance system 'domestic spinsters' who stayed at home to care for elderly parents. Beveridge's serious attempts to adapt the social security system to the specific needs of women as well as those of men very largely failed. Conventional assumptions and practices concerning gender roles were hard to break, even by an influential man writing an otherwise highly influential Report.[24]

The social security system after the war, not very surprisingly – since social welfare regimes express prevailing social norms – appeared to reinforce conventional gender roles, family relationships and norms of behaviour, which it took for granted.

They did not succeed in preserving them wholly. The post-war period saw a rise in divorce rates and, especially in the 1980s and 1990s, a radical change in household forms, though not in the relative incomes in the paid labour market of female single parents.

For reasons of economy post-war pensions were set at lower levels than Beveridge had recommended. This did not prevent the practice of retirement at ages 60 or 65 spreading with un-precedented rapidity. For the first time, during the 1950s, it became the norm among manual, mainly male, workers, despite efforts by the government to prevent it because of the post-war labour shortage.[25]

A consequence of the low level of pensions was that very large numbers of old people (a majority of them female) continued to live in poverty after the war. For all Beveridge's good intentions the means test was never abolished for the poorest. They had still to supplement the insurance pension with means-tested National Assistance and its successors.

Local social service agencies and social workers appear to have taken more interest in the needs of older people after the war. Before the war mothers and children seem to have been a greater focus of concern. The change may have come about partly because surveys at the beginning of the war had shown many old people to be living in conditions far more appalling than had been realised.[26] Also, a general panic about the effects of the ageing of British society – which began in the 1930s – still raged in the later 1940s, despite an upturn in the birthrate.[27] This helped focus attention on old people as a problem group from the later 1930s. Geriatrics – considered as a serious medical specialism – was pioneered in Britain by a female doctor, Marjorie Warren.[28] Services originally invented by women to meet the needs of mothers and infants – such as health visitors, 'home helps' and district nurses – were increasingly used by older people, who still showed a strong preference for living independently in their own homes until as late an age as possible. It was a new phase in a long tradition of women caring for old people in the community on behalf of that community.

There seemed also to have been little change over time in customary assumptions and in the practice of family responsibility for old people. The Poor Law Act 1930 restated the principles of the 1601 Poor Law:

It should be the duty of the father, grandfather, mother, grandmother, husband or child of a poor, old, blind, lame or impotent person, or other poor person, not able to work, if possessed of sufficient means, to relieve and maintain that person.

But the authorities appeared reluctant once again to enforce such responsibility, when families could afford to observe it only with difficulty; and families appear still to have acknowledged their responsibility voluntarily whenever they were able. The obligation to do so was abolished in 1946.

CONCLUSION

Over the period from the mid-nineteenth to the mid-twentieth centuries 'old people' were increasingly clearly defined as a distinctive social group, and the aged poor as a marginalised social group. Most of this group was female and a gender analysis – in particular the conception of the welfare state as patriarchal – has value in drawing our attention to certain aspects of the experience and treatment of old people; but it is not adequate on its own to explain many features of that experience. Patriarchy was one of the taken-for-granted assumptions in policy-making, but its influence could be overridden by other assumptions and priorities. In particular it needs to be supplemented by another set of theories and concepts sensitive to age as another primary division in society, alongside class, gender and race, attentive to what old men and old women have in common, as mediated by class and race, as well as what separates them. Gender must be used in conjunction with other categories to reach a fuller understanding of policy change or of wider socio-economic changes.

NOTES

1 Patricia Hollis, *Ladies Elect: Women in English Local Government, 1865–1914*, Oxford, Oxford University Press, 1987.
2 Frank Prochaska, *Women and Philanthropy in Nineteenth Century England*, Oxford, Oxford University Press, 1980.
3 E. A. Wrigley and R. S. Schofield, *The Population History of England, 1541–1871*, Cambridge, Cambridge University Press, 1989, pp. 528–9.
4 Paul Slack, *The English Poor Law 1531–1782*, London, Macmillan, 1990.

5 Much of the research on which these statements are based is referred to and summarised in the 'Introduction' to Margaret Pelling and R. M. Smith (eds), *Life, Death and the Elderly: Historical Perspectives*, London, Routledge, 1991.

6 Pelling and Smith, *Life*.

7 Slack, *English Poor Law*, and *Poverty and Policy in Tudor and Stuart England*, London, Longman, 1988.

8 M. Barker-Read, 'The Treatment of the Aged Poor in Five Selected West Kent Parishes from Settlement to Speenhamland (1662–1797)', PhD thesis, Open University, 1988.

9 Pat Thane, 'Non-contributory versus Insurance Pensions,1878-1908', in Pat Thane (ed.), *The Origins of British Social Policy*, London, Croom Helm, 1978, pp. 84–106.

10 D. Thomson, 'The Welfare of the Elderly in the Past: A Family or Community Responsibility?', in Pelling and Smith (eds), *Life*, pp. 194–221.

11 Leslie Hannah, *Inventing Retirement: The Development of Occupational Pensions in Britain*, Cambridge, Cambridge University Press, 1986.

12 M. Anderson 'The Emergence of the Modern Life Cycle in Britain', *Social History*, 1985, vol. 10, p. 85.

13 J. Fogerty, 'Growing Old in England 1878–1948', PhD dissertation, Australian National University, 1992, p. 8; Paul Johnson, 'The Employment and Retirement of Older Men in England and Wales, 1881–1981', *Economic History Review*, vol. XLVII, no. 1, February 1994.

14 Fogerty, 'Growing Old'.

15 This campaign is described in Thane, 'Non-contributory'.

16 Thane, 'Non-contributory', p. 186.

17 Christoph Conrad, 'The Emergence of Modern Retirement: Germany in an International Comparison (1850–1960)', *Population. An English Selection*, 1991, vol. 3, pp. 171–200.

18 A. Wilson and G. S. Mackay, *Old Age Pensions: An Historical and Critical Study*, Oxford, Oxford University Press, 1941, p. 104.

19 Wilson and Mackay, *Old Age*, p. 134.

20 They were contributory for those in the insurance system.

21 Wilson and Mackay, *Old Age*, p. 134.

22 Widows, Orphans and Old Age Contributory Pensions Act 1925; Annual Accounts 1927–39, *Parliamentary Papers*, annually.

23 Carol Miller, 'Lobbying the League: Women's International Organisations and the League of Nations', DPhil thesis, University of Oxford, 1992.

24 José Harris, *William Beveridge*, Oxford, Oxford University Press, 1977, pp. 402–4.

25 Sarah Harper and Pat Thane, 'The Consolidation of 'Old Age' as a Phase of Life, 1945–65', in M. Jeffreys (ed.), *Growing Old in the Twentieth Century*, London, Routledge, 1989, pp. 43–61.

26 Fogerty, 'Growing Old'.

27 Pat Thane, 'The Debate on the Declining Birth-rate in Britain: the

"Menace" of an Ageing Population, 1920s–1950s', *Continuity and Change*, 1990, vol. 5, no. 2, pp. 283–305.

28 Pat Thane, 'Geriatrics', in W. Bynum and R. Porter (eds), *Companion Encyclopedia of the History of Medicine*, London, Routledge, 1993, vol. 2, pp. 1092–1118.

Chapter 9

Gender and welfare in the late nineteenth and early twentieth centuries

Jane Lewis

THE SIGNIFICANCE OF GENDER

In the historiography of welfare provision, gender has played little part, which is in large measure the result of the small amount of attention paid to the family as an element in the 'mixed economy of welfare'. For example, in Richard Titmuss' classic framework for understanding the dimensions of welfare he analysed three aspects: occupational welfare, fiscal welfare and state services and transfers. In this framework there was no mention of the family or the voluntary sector as providers of welfare and no mention of gender as an important variable, only social class was consid-ered in the analysis of access to welfare and outcomes of social provision.[1] Yet as Ann Oakley has suggested: 'to talk of welfare was and is to make assumptions about the roles of men and women which, if challenged, call into question the very notion of social welfare itself'.[2]

The early literature on women and welfare tended to focus on women as 'victims' of the welfare system and to emphasise the extent to which social policies represented 'the state organisation of domestic life',[3] or a form of 'public patriarchy' (this term was used first in early Scandinavian feminist analyses).[4] This focus has tended to stress the extent to which state welfare policies have been imposed on women and have been extremely valuable in highlighting the importance of assumptions regarding the way in which the family works, especially in respect of the presence of a 'male breadwinner', and hence for understanding the way in which women are treated as clients of welfare systems. Assumptions as to the existence of a male breadwinner and female and child dependants has meant, first, that women's contributions to welfare, both paid and unpaid, have not received the recognition that is their due and hence women have received less by way of benefits; and, second, that women's needs have tended to be defined in terms of motherhood as a social function rather than individually.

The idea of 'public patriarchy' has also served to capture the extent to which the increase in women's paid labour, in the period after World War II, and especially in the case of married women, has been largely in the service of the welfare state. In other words, women's traditional work of caring has to some extent moved into the public world of paid labour. More recent feminist analysis of the family in relation to social policies has sought to emphasise both that it is all too easy to make assumptions about family form and that 'the family' actually consists of men, women and children, it being women who continue to provide the majority of the informal care.[5]

However, what is arguably central to an analysis of women and welfare are the relationships between women as providers of welfare and women as clients of the welfare system, and between women as paid providers of welfare and unpaid providers. The use of gender, understood as a fundamental organising principle in society,[6] is crucial to a more general understanding of welfare systems. Access to resources of all kinds – education, income and work – has been and is profoundly gendered, as are the concepts central to the analysis of social policies, e.g. citizenship and inequality. Women cannot simply be 'added-on' to an analysis of welfare systems. An approach that focuses on the 'gendered divisions of welfare' means that it is possible to appreciate how, for example, governments may at one and the same time adhere to the view that the family should consist of two parents and children, with men playing the role of breadwinners and women acting primarily as carers, and yet step in, under strict conditions, to fill the place of the male breadwinner in lone mother families, thus permitting the transformation of the family form. Or, how women's work in terms of making meals for school children may take place in the home or under the auspices of a voluntary society at the turn of the century, moving into the world of paid labour in the service of the welfare state in the second half of the twentieth century, but always remaining women's work. Broadly speaking, there are, in modern welfare states, three major sources of income for women: men, the labour market and the state and during the twentieth century there has been a major shift towards increased dependence on the labour market for married women and for single women without children, and towards dependence on the state for lone women with children. But because of the gendered division of both paid and unpaid work, married women continue to rely on both wages and husbands for support and single women on wages and the state. It therefore becomes not so much a question of deciding whether state welfare in particular has been good or bad for women, but of examining the interplay in welfare systems that have often been pulling in different directions while still serving to preserve gender divisions.

In this chapter I shall address the position of women as clients of welfare regimes and as providers of welfare. Crucially for women, welfare has historically been synonymous with giving, in the form of paid and unpaid caring work, just as much as with taking from the state. The way in which women are positioned as clients and providers has much to do with the nature of the particular welfare regime and it is to a consideration of this in late nineteenth- and early twentieth-century Britain that I turn first.

GENDER AND WELFARE REGIMES

Recent comparative work on modern welfare states has emphasised the importance of the relationship between state and economy, and in particular between work and welfare.[7] Work is defined as paid work and welfare as policies that permit, encourage or discourage the decommodification of labour. While this represents a substantial advance on the older literature which focused only on the comparative development of policies of social amelioration,[8] it misses two of the central issues in the structuring of welfare regimes: first, the problem of valuing the unpaid work that is done primarily by women in providing welfare, mainly within the family, and in securing those providers' social entitlements. The crucial relationship is not just between paid work and welfare, but as Peter Taylor Gooby recently remarked, between paid work, unpaid work and welfare,[9] and it is particularly important for understanding women's position as clients in welfare systems. Second, the recent literature on modern welfare regimes has tended to pay insufficient attention to the importance of the mixed economy of welfare provision, whereby the state, the voluntary sector, the family and the market have all played their parts, the importance of which has shifted over time (although informal provision through the family has remained remarkably constant). The nature of the mixed economy of welfare has proved important historically for understanding how women's contribution as providers of welfare has been elicited.

The relationship between paid work, unpaid work and welfare is gendered in that while it is possible to argue that the divisions in paid work have substantially diminished, to the extent that greater numbers of women have entered the labour market (although not with regard to pay, status and hours), all the evidence suggests that the division of unpaid work has remained substantially the same.[10] Thus concepts such as 'decommodification' or 'dependency' have a gendered meaning that is rarely acknowledged. While Esping Andersen writes of decommodification as a necessary prerequisite for workers' political mobilisation, the worker he has in mind is male and his mobilisation may depend as much on unpaid female household labour as on state policies. Decommodification for women via the development of social security systems is likely to result in their carrying out unpaid caring work; in other words 'welfare dependency' on the part of adult women is likely to result in the greater independence of another person, young or old. The unequal division of unpaid work thus blurs the dichotomous divisions between dependent and independent, commodified and decommodified.

As Kolberg has noted, the interface between the private in the sense of the informal provision of welfare, the market and the state has not been subjected to close analysis.[11] Just as informal care was absent from Titmuss' division of welfare in 1963, so it is just as absent from more recent categorisations.[12] In the work of Esping Andersen, or of Leibfried, women disappear from the analysis when they disappear from labour markets.[13] Yet consideration of the private/domestic is crucial to any understanding of women's position because historically women have typically gained welfare entitlements by virtue of their dependent status within the family as wives, the justification being a division of labour perceived to follow 'naturally' on their capacity for motherhood. Women have thus tended to make contributions and draw benefits via their husbands in accordance with assumptions regarding the existence of the male-breadwinner family model.[14] Furthermore, in welfare regimes such as that of Britain (and the

United States), where the social security system has developed a dual insurance/assistance model, this in and of itself tends to be gendered, with first-class (insurance) benefits going mainly to men and second-class (welfare/assistance) benefits to women.[15] Thus the 1911 national unemployment insurance legislation covered those trades in which mainly skilled, male workers were employed.

The development of modern welfare states in the late nineteenth and early twentieth centuries coincided with the period when the boundary between the public world of paid work and political participation and the private domain of the family was strongest in both the prescriptive literature and in reality, at least for middle-class women. In its ideal form the male-breadwinner model prescribed breadwinning for men and caring/homemaking for women. It was part of a much larger gendered division between public and private that informed the work of philosophers after Locke, and was taken as one of the measures of a civilised society by late nineteenth-century social theorists such as Herbert Spencer. Working within an evolutionary framework, Spencer argued that society was 'progressing' towards a position whereby all women would be able to stay at home in their 'natural' sphere. While it may be argued that his was a shared ideal – between men and women, employees and employers and the state[16] – it is important to note that it was never completely achieved. The male-breadwinner model operated most fully for late-nineteenth-century middle-class women in a few industrialised countries. Working-class women have always engaged in paid labour to some degree.

In reality, as Sokoloff and Pateman have each insisted, the public and private spheres have been, and are, intimately interrelated rather than separated.[17] Not least as a provider of welfare the family has been central to civil society, rather than separate from it. Over time the boundary between public and private has been redrawn at the level of prescription. For example, in English the phrase 'working mother' entered the language during and after World War II, but wage earning was always deemed a secondary activity for women. Given that in modern societies independence derives primarily from wage earning,[18] the assumption that women were located mainly in the private sphere supported by a male breadwinner also meant that women have only been partially individualised. In regard to social policies, the liberal dilemma first described by Okin, whereby individuals in fact meant male heads of families, has persisted.[19] Modern welfare regimes have all subscribed to some degree to the idea of a male breadwinner model, although its persistence in the late twentieth century has varied considerably between countries.

In regard to women as providers of welfare, their position has been affected greatly by the nature of the mixed economy of welfare. Informal provision in the family has remained remarkably constant. Its contribution was considered crucial by the nineteenth-century voluntary sector, indeed a large part of voluntary action was directed towards eliciting the kind of behaviour from the adult members of poor families that would secure their self-maintenance and the health and welfare of their children. The shift in the balance within the mixed economy away from the voluntary sector and towards a much larger role for the state during the twentieth century has often been accompanied by the charge that government usurped the role of the family (and the voluntary sector), providing institutional care for the elderly, and day care and education for children.[20] Many writers have pointed out that there is little evidence of the family doing less, for example, the percentage of elderly people in institutions has been remarkably stable throughout the twentieth century,[21] and while schools and clinics have taken on many of the responsibilities in respect of children, the family has found new tasks especially in regard to fostering the emotional development of children and in playing a complementary role to the school in securing their intellectual development through, for example, supervising homework.

While the level of the family's contribution has not changed markedly, the balance between the voluntary and the statutory sector has, and this has had a significant impact on women's contribution as providers of welfare. The size of the voluntary sector in the late nineteenth century is hard to measure. Humphreys has argued that any claim that charity provided more in relief to the poor than the poor law must be treated with suspicion, but if the work of the medical charities and philanthropic public works are taken into consideration then charity may be said to have bulked larger than the state in terms of social provision.[22] There is certainly plenty of evidence that late Victorian middle-class households made substantial contributions to charity; in the 1890s it has been estimated that on average they spent a larger share of their income on charity than on any item in their budget except food.[23]

As Pat Thane has observed, voluntarism in the nineteenth century was not the fortuitous corollary of a limited state, but was integral to the conceptualisation of that state.[24] Unlike continental European states, Britain had a relatively small central bureaucracy. Its central government institutions were efficient, but the aim of late-nineteenth-century political leaders was to provide a framework in which individuals were free and self-governing. A set of rules and guidelines were provided and were designed to enable society to run itself.[25] Furthermore, at the turn of the century social provision was locally financed and locally administered. Social policies were only becoming matters of 'high politics' in the period 1870–1914, and the New Liberal welfare reforms of 1906–1914 used taxation as a social instrument for the first time to provide nationally determined programmes of health and sickness insurance and of old age pensions.

The fact that social provision was local at the turn of the century means that it was in some ways easier for a measure of welfare pluralism to exist, and for the voluntary sector in particular to play a large part. The balance between the voluntary and the statutory sectors shifted as ideas about the scope of central government's activity changed. The early twentieth century saw the rise of ideas about 'national efficiency', the notion of the importance of securing a healthy population (above all in the wake of debate about the débâcle of the Boer War), together with other social services (such as education), that could be said to contribute towards social investment. Social provision, such as the old age pension, was also envisaged as moderating the effects of increased international industrial competition on the labour force. While women's voluntary action was perceived as a legitimate extension of their role in the family, employment in the service of the state was not. Thus the early twentieth century shift in the balance of welfare provision from the voluntary sector to the state had profound implications for female providers of welfare.

WOMEN AS CLIENTS

Women's position as clients in the British welfare regime has been determined in large measure by the extent to which assumptions regarding the existence of a male-breadwinner model family have underpinned both charitable and state social provision. In its pure form, the male-breadwinner model predicts that married women will not engage in paid work, but rather will undertake the work of caring (for children and other dependants) at home without public support, and that they will be subordinated to their husbands for the purposes of social security entitlements and tax. In reality, such a model has never existed. Charles Booth's social survey of London showed that 30 per cent of the population was unable to rely on a man's wage in 1889, while Bowley estimated in 1921 that only 41 per cent of working-class families were dependent on a man's wage alone. Nevertheless, it was broadly accepted that the male-breadwinner model 'ought' to characterise the way families organised themselves. Working women showed as little enthusiasm for a job outside the home as policy-makers. During a period in which working-class women underwent frequent pregnancy and engaged in hard household labour, women who had to undertake paid work were likely to be pitied.[26] However, when policy-makers used the idea of the male-breadwinner model family to underpin their legislative proposals they translated an 'ought' into an 'is' with adverse effects for women.

In line with the dominant turn-of-the-century view of gender roles in the family and their link to social stability and welfare, Helen Bosanquet, a leading member of the Charity Organisation Society, argued that the 'stable family' with its male breadwinner was 'the only known way of ensuring with an approach to success, that one generation will exert itself in the interests and for the sake of another'. Evidence of family failure was twofold: first, the physical welfare of children measured by indices such as the incidence of child neglect and the infant mortality rate, and, second, the number of families seeking relief under the poor law. Men were suspected of laziness and unwillingness to shoulder the responsibility for providing for women and children. The economist, F. Y. Edgeworth, quoted approvingly the comment that a social worker made in 1908, to the effect that 'if the husband got out of work, the only thing the wife should do is sit down and cry, because if she did anything else he would remain out of work'.[27] Women were held responsible for the management of households and the welfare of children, but commentators at the turn of the century tended to show more sympathy for working-class wives, regarding them for the most part as well-meaning but ignorant and often oppressed by selfish husbands. Most of the effort expended by charity and the state, working through social workers and later health visitors and infant welfare clinics, was directed at working-class mothers.

The leaders in the world of charity devoted most of their attention to trying to make sure that the behaviour of working-class families conformed to the prescriptions of the male-breadwinner model. Lasting reform, they believed, could only be achieved by changing people. Thus, they placed their faith in social workers who would work with individuals, usually mothers, and their families to change their habits, build up their characters and give new purpose to their lives. Individual social work was conceived of as a form of education and the means of promoting economic independence and fully participative citizens.

Personal social service was usually called 'friendly visiting' in the late nineteenth century. It meant, in theory at least, the careful and sympathetic investigation of the applicant's case and the formulation of a plan of treatment. Friendly visitors were assigned families and were told 'to befriend, aid and elevate' the people they visited.[28] The first lesson for friendly visitors was to befriend the poor, rather than to approach them as people in need of assistance. This immediately called into question the practice of mixing relief with visiting, because, as Octavia Hill put it, 'doles darkened friendship'.[29] Hill instructed visitors that they should first give 'sympathetic, imaginative consideration' to the case to see what the causes of the problem were : 'he is worth no one's money; he is ill and needs cure; or he is idle or ignorant, or bad tempered, and needs – my friends, what does he need?'[30] She warned that it was never easy to help a member of one's own family and that the difficulties would be greater still when dealing with strangers, but that it would help the visitor if she tried to deal with the poor as she would a family member. Too much help and the person needing assistance would become dependent, too little and he would lose hope. The main aim of the visitor was to ensure that men undertook regular labour, supported their families and saved for periods of misfortune, and that women kept houses and children clean and managed the household budget. (See also Chapter 4.)

It is easy to be scornful of Hill's injunction to visitors to befriend the poor. At the end of the day, the aim of the visitor was to bring about change in the households she visited. As Hill put it: 'my only notion of reform is that of living side by side with people, till all that one believes becomes clear to them'.[31] This kind of social action was 'detailed', and consisted of 'infinitesimally small actions' designed to change the way in which the poor behaved.[32] In friendly visiting, the visitor was supposed to gain the trust of the working-class wife and mother and then lead by example. But in the end the visitor was expected to try to get poor families to see the virtues of middle-class ways, values and culture. Nevertheless, working-class women were not necessarily antagonistic to the work of visitors. Hannah Mitchell, a working-class suffragist, recorded in her autobiography that she wished there had been some advice available to her when her children had been young.[33] And Pat Thane has argued that working-class men and women in the early part of the century wanted non-stigmatising and non-intrusive welfare provision to tide them over periods of misfortune.[34]

Leading opinion within the world of charity believed that there was little material aid that could be offered the family that would not damage family responsibility and subvert character. By offering old age pensions, or national insurance against sickness and unemployment, state intervention was condemned as likely to undermine character, whereas volunteer social workers, suitably trained, would serve to strengthen character and deepen the ties of voluntary obligation within the community. Achieving social change by changing habits was acknowledged to be an inordinately slow business, but it was felt to be the only sure route to permanent improvement. One Charity Organisation Society member, Joseph Lee, described the society's opposition to school meals as a crucial last stand: 'outlying territory we can abandon, but here our citadel is reached. If we cannot defend this wall we might as well surrender'.[35]

However, substantial numbers of politicians were also perturbed by the idea that the state might subvert family responsibility, but were convinced by arguments put forward from all points on the political spectrum that it was 'increasingly difficult to accept the view that the great forces of the state are only to be at the service of the pauper, the lunatic, and the criminal'.[36] Nonetheless, the legislators were cautious. In the case of school meals, parents were expected to contribute to the costs and the school attendance officer was usually given the task of assessing means. When school medical inspection was introduced in 1907, parents (usually mothers) were advised what was wrong with their children, but were not provided with access to treatment.

Anna Martin, a settlement worker, complained that without the provision of treatment school medical inspection became an injunction to 'make bricks without straw', and this rested particularly harshly on mothers.[37]

Notwithstanding the concern about high infant mortality rates, national health insurance, introduced in 1911, covered only wage earners and not dependants, which again meant that fathers were expected to exercise their obligation to maintain. Nor did unemployment insurance, also introduced in 1911 cover women and children, unless the woman was in full-time insurable employment (only 10 per cent were so placed). As the Fabian Women's Group pointed out, contributory insurance was bound to reflect the existing economic position of women and divide them into those living as their husbands' dependants and those living as economically-independent individuals.[38] In 1911 the Women's Industrial Council (a group of primarily middle-class women who devoted themselves to the investigation of working women's problems) went so far as to suggest that such a form of provision was inappropriate for women, and merely intensified the 'regrettable tendency to consider the work of a wife and mother in her home of no money value'.[39]

Women who were covered by national insurance found that they tended to be submitted to strict surveillance by national health insurance visitors because of the unexpectedly large number of sickness claims. Married women were thought to be particularly likely to abuse the system because of the temptation to stay at home to catch up with housework.[40] Pregnancy also posed difficulties to those administering health insurance, which showed how difficult it was for state welfare policies to treat women as workers and mothers. Married women were always treated as a class apart for insurance purposes and in 1932 they found their health insurance benefits cut because of the high risk they represented, even though no other group with excessive claims (for example, miners) was singled out for similar treatment. Men, on the other hand, were granted dependants' benefits under national insurance in 1922, plus the married man's tax allowance from 1919, on the assumption that a man supporting a wife needed additional tax relief (in fact the allowance was paid to all men regardless of whether or not their wives went out to work).

On the whole, the new forms of insurance provision were designed for the regularly employed male worker. Women in need of material help were often forced to rely on the poor law if they could not secure help from charity. The late-nineteenth and early-twentieth-century poor law found it very difficult to decide how to treat women who were without husbands but who had children – the widow, the deserted wife and the unmarried mother. Were they to be regarded as mothers or as workers? Treatment varied considerably from place to place. A Local Government Board circular of 1871 had advised local Boards of Guardians that outdoor relief should not be granted to the able-bodied widow with one child and in cases where there was more than one child the widow's need should be tested by offering to take the children into the workhouse rather than give her outdoor relief. Deserted wives were regarded with even more suspicion than widows and it was recommended that they be denied any help for twelve months to ensure that they were not 'colluding' with their husbands to defraud the authorities. Unmarried mothers were treated most harshly of all because of the danger posed by their immoral behaviour.[41] The 1909 Royal Commission on the Poor Laws found that for widows the first recommendation of 1871 was generally observed, in other words women without breadwinners were expected to become breadwinners themselves. However, because outdoor relief was cheaper than taking children into the workhouse, many guardians were prepared to give supplementary outdoor relief to lone mothers.[42]

Running parallel to the concern to preserve and promote the working-class husband's obligation to maintain and the wife's primary duty as unpaid homemaker and carer was suspicion of married women's employment. At the 1906 National Conference on Infant Mortality, John Burns, the President of the Local Government Board, called for stringent restrictions on all married women's work.[43] Yet little protection was offered to the married woman as worker; Britain failed to implement paid maternity leave and never ratified the International Labour Organisation's Washington Convention provision for six weeks paid leave.[44] The concern was not so much to maximise the welfare of working women as mothers, as to minimise their labour market participation. The most stringent limitations of women's work opportunities were imposed in the professions, where a 'marriage bar' was introduced during the 1920s. The 1919 Treasury Committee on recruitment to the civil service after the war stated firmly that family responsibilities were incompatible with devotion to public service.[45] During the inter-war years, national insurance provided a means of channelling women into 'suitable' work. Women applying for benefit under the Unemployment Insurance Acts could be required to train as domestic servants, and after 1931, under the Anomalies Act, married women who left the labour force for whatever reason were effectively assumed to have retired. (See also Chapter 3.)

Assumptions regarding the male-breadwinner family model proved extremely long-lived when it came to the principles underpinning state welfare provision. Under the post-war Beveridgean settlement, women continued to be treated as dependants for the purposes of social security entitlements. (See also Chapters 3 and 8.) Beveridge wrote at length of the importance of women's role as wives and mothers in ensuring the continuance of the British race (at a time of fears about population decline) and insisted on marriage as a 'partnership' rather than a patriarchal relationship.[46] It was, however, a partnership in which the parties were to be equal but different. Hence women were defined as wives and mothers and therefore as dependent on a male wage. Married women were accordingly invited to take the 'married women's option' paying less by way of contributions and collecting less in benefits. The married women's option was not abandoned until the middle of the 1970s with the passing of equal opportunities legislation.

WOMEN AS PROVIDERS

Recent work, by historians and sociologists interested in the comparative development of social provision, has sought to address gender and has done so by highlighting the part played by women and the importance of gender issues in the building of welfare states.[47] This has introduced a further dimension to the debate between those seeking to revise the view that welfare states emerged as part of the process of modernisation by emphasising the importance of social class, and the initiatives of bureaucrats, professionals or employers.[48]

The new work on gender and the origins of welfare states has stressed women's role as actors in providing welfare from an early stage, chiefly via voluntary organisations, and has labelled this action 'social maternalist politics'. Kathryn Kish Sklar has gone so far as to argue that, in the United States, women's social activism served as a surrogate for working-class social-welfare activism.[49] Koven and Michel have argued for the substantial influence of women in shaping welfare states in Britain as well as the USA, suggesting that this was possible because these states were 'weak', as opposed to the 'strong' states of Germany or France, where women's influence was weaker.[50] This argument is somewhat at odds with that of Skocpol and Ritter, who emphasise the extent to which all European, including British, early welfare legislation was paternalist compared to the USA, where mothers' pensions and protective labour legislation were the most common forms of intervention at state level.[51] The 1906 New Liberal welfare reforms provided national insurance cover for primarily male workers, while in the USA programmes for women directed by women came into being.

What both sets of arguments have in common is a case for women's agency in the building of welfare states. But agency must be contextualised. In many respects both Koven and Michel and Skocpol and Ritter are right. The former rightly insist on the importance of British women's voluntary action, which Skocpol and Ritter tend to miss. However, the latter are right to maintain that women did not exert much influence on the core elements of Edwardian state welfare legislation, that is old age pensions and national insurance. Koven and Michel tend to elide a commitment to primarily voluntary social action with the building of state welfare because they judge the British state to have been 'weak'. But it is more accurate to see central government keeping a firm hold on key activities of state and delegating functions considered less essential to local authorities and voluntary organisations.[52] For women as providers of welfare the crucial point is that until the end of the first decade of the twentieth century the nature of the mixed economy of welfare was tilted firmly in favour of the voluntary sector and local government.

British women were able to act because of the specific nature of the mixed economy of welfare at the turn of the century which was tilted firmly in favour of the voluntary sector and local government. Not only were the voluntary sector and local government considered appropriate places for women to work, but contemporary social thought highlighted the importance of the particular kind of work – personal social work – that women did at the local level. As the balance of the mixed economy of welfare shifted in favour of a centralised welfare system and the philosophy of welfare changed, such that structural change came to be seen as more important than changing the habits and behaviour of individuals, so women's influence decreased. Women were largely shut out from any influential positions in respect of state welfare from the introduction of national insurance through to the legislation of the post-war Labour government. The closest that women got to the administration of the national insurance scheme was to serve as sickness visitors to check on malingerers.

Women were very active in local government, as poor law guardians, members of boards of education and increasingly as councillors. Both Patricia Hollis and, for the USA, Paula Baker have argued that, using the language of separate spheres, women succeeded in 'domesticating' politics.[53] Even if they were implicated in the administration of a poor-relief system that conferred considerable stigma on recipients, it is argued that women succeeded in 'humanising' important aspects of that system, especially in regard to the regime of workhouses. Hollis has contended that 'women remade the workhouse' by the attention they gave to detail and to the individual inmates.[54] Similarly, women who were elected to school boards tended to make the welfare of children their special concern. For example, in Bradford Margaret McMillan worked to secure school baths in the 1890s, although not all intervention on the part of women was necessarily progressive. As a member of the Chesterfield School Board in 1898, Violet Markham fought to retain school fees because of her belief in the importance of the father's obligation to maintain.

Women and men across the political spectrum, and both those in favour of and against votes for women, were able to support female social action at the local level. But there is little evidence of women's activity at the national level, where their right to political citizenship was not recognised. One of the few positions in the civil service to which women gained access was that of factory inspector, after a long campaign stressing the importance of this for the full implementation of protective labour legislation. As social policy issues became matters of high politics in the period 1870-1914, so women were faced with the decision whether to try to move with them. Anti-suffragists like Mrs Humphry Ward, who founded the Women's Local Government Association, decided against because national politics were in the main imperial politics and outside women's sphere. But someone like Beatrice Webb changed her mind about the desirability of the vote as it became clear that social questions were becoming national questions. Women were only able to 'domesticate the public' sphere within certain well-defined limits. Local government and the voluntary sector were conceptualised as extensions of family and neighbourhood, whereas national politics and policy-making were not. Women made the transition from unpaid voluntary visitor to paid health visitor and social worker in the employ of local government, but very rarely to policy-making positions in the civil service.

Women's political and administrative weakness in the new welfare apparatus of the early-twentieth-century state is clearly demonstrated in the fate of feminist arguments for family allowances between 1918 and 1944.[55] Feminists conceived of allowances as a way first of rewarding women's unpaid caring work. In the initial proposal in 1918, an allowance for the mother was included as well as for children. But it also sought to achieve equality in wages. If women and children were receiving a social wage, male workers would no longer be able to bargain for a family wage. As Susan Pedersen has traced, the claim was defeated by the power of three oppositional discourses: first, social scientists arguing that women could not be said to have dependants; second, Labour Party men and male trade unionists who argued for the family wage to keep up male wages, often revealing in the process the way in which the responsibility for maintaining a family was perceived as an emblem of masculinity; and, third, civil servants who denied that the support of motherhood should be the direct concern of government.[56] The eventual 1944 legislation was designed primarily to keep down wage-push inflation.[57]

The vast majority of women providers of welfare worked in the voluntary sector and through the family. Of course, many social programmes such as school meals and child and maternal welfare centres were 'pioneered' by voluntary organisations and were taken over by the state in the later Edwardian period and during World War I. But given the gendered division of labour in the voluntary sector, whereby women did most of the friendly visiting or social work and men ran the committees,[58] women were not likely to achieve influential positions in what became state-run services. There is also a more general issue as to how porous boundaries actually were between the voluntary and statutory sectors. The Charity Organisation Society worked according to a notion of an explicit division between the territory of charity and that of the state; the 'pioneer' model of relationships between the two sectors did not universally apply.

Nevertheless, the work women did perform as mainly volunteer social workers was accorded great importance because it was believed that it represented the way to achieve social change. The job of the female visitor was pivotal; she had the task of going into homes and restoring the will of family members to become independent and self-supporting. Indeed, social work was perceived to have a significance at the turn of the century that it has never achieved since. As the balance in the mixed economy of welfare shifted towards the state provision of a national minimum level of material welfare, so social work became a residual activity.

Women did play a major role in social provision at the turn of the century outside the confines of the state. But it is difficult to say how they conceptualised their contribution. The recent literature on gender and the origins of welfare states has portrayed them as 'maternalists', defined by Skocpol in terms of extending domestic ideals into public life. As we have seen, in the British context this meant securing change in working-class families by promoting middle-class notions of proper breadwinning behaviour for men and good housekeeping and childcare standards for women. This does not mean that there was not substantial sympathy for the lot of poor women on the part of the visitors or that poor women did not want much of the help that was offered, but it is far from clear how the definition of maternalism differs from paternalism. Nor is it clear that the sole inspiration for these women's work was maternalist in the sense of wishing to promote the welfare of all mothers and children. Rather, women's social action was often part and parcel of middle-class women's ideas about the duties of citizenship.[59] The language of duty and the injunction to serve was ubiquitous for men and women, but it was gendered in its implications – women served via their families and the performance of voluntary social work while men entered the public world of work and politics.

Hollis, Koven and Michel have argued that women were able to use the language of separate spheres to their advantage. But while women were successful in claiming a narrow territory of social intervention, the long-term implications were less appealing. Women became identified with a specific form of social provision which made them both the agents and the objects of reform.[60] The notion of 'women's mission to women' relied on the idea that women were both cause and cure of social ills, something that has persisted through twentieth-century debates about juvenile delinquency and lone parenthood.

CONCLUSION

Welfare is and has been gendered in complex ways. This chapter has sought to illustrate but two of these: the extent to which assumptions regarding family form and the role of adult family members informed both voluntary and legislative efforts in the late nineteenth and the first half of the twentieth centuries; and the extent to which women were important as providers of welfare not just in their families but also in the voluntary sector at the turn of the century. But it is important that any consideration of gender and welfare be contextualised. Thus it will not do to see policies based on assumptions regarding the male-breadwinner model as a simple conspiracy against women. Many women at the turn of the century had good reason to share the male-breadwinner model as an ideal, even if its reality eluded them. What is interesting is to trace the moment at which the model ceased to be an ideal for women. After that point policies based on it were severely out-of-step with female opinion. In all probability, this occurred after the more effective control of fertility and the expansion of married women's labour market participation which occurred after World War II. Similarly, women's position as providers of welfare must be contextualised. It is inadequate to explain their actions in terms of 'maternalism' without due attention both to other kinds of motivation, whether the search for adventure or the fulfilment of citizenship obligations, and to the particular nature of the mixed economy of welfare that made their considerable contribution possible at the turn of the century. Welfare regimes have been profoundly gendered, but we are only beginning – as in the discussions in this volume – to delineate how.

NOTES

1 R. M. Titmuss, 'The Social Division of Welfare', in R. M. Titmuss, *Essays on the Welfare State*, London, Allen & Unwin, 1963.

2　A. Oakley, 'Social Welfare and the Position of Women. Titmuss Memorial Lecture', Hebrew University of Jerusalem, 18 May 1986.
3　E. Wilson, *Women and the Welfare State*, London, Tavistock, 1977.
4　B. Siim, 'The Scandinavian Welfare States – Towards Sexual Equality or a new Kind of Male Domination?', *Acta Sociologica*, 1987, vol. 30, nos 3/4.
5　J. Finch and D. Groves (eds), *A Labour of Love. Women, Work and Caring*, London, Routledge & Kegan Paul, 1983.
6　J. Scott, *Gender and the Politics of History*, New York, Columbia University Press, 1987.
7　G. Esping Andersen, *The Three Worlds of Welfare Capitalism*, Cambridge, Polity Press, 1990.
8　H. L. Wilensky and C. N. Lebaux, *Industrial Society and Social Welfare*, New York, The Free Press, 1965.
9　P. Taylor Gooby, 'Welfare State Regimes and Welfare Citizenship', *Journal of European Social Policy*, 1965, vol. 1, no. 2.
10　L. Morris, *The Workings of the Household. A US–UK Comparison*, Cambridge, Polity Press, 1965.
11　J. E. Kolberg, 'The Gender Dimension of the Welfare State', *International Journal of Sociology*, 1991, vol. 21, no. 2.
12　M. Langan and I. Ostner, 'Gender and Welfare', in G. Room (ed.), *Towards a European Welfare State*? Bristol, School for Advanced Urban Studies, 1991.
13　S. Leibfried, 'Towards a European Welfare State? On the Integration Potentials of Poverty Regimes in the EC', Working Paper, Bremen University, 1991.
14　H. Land, 'The Family Wage', *Feminist Review*, 1980, vol. 6.
15　L. Gordon (ed.), *Women, The State and Welfare*, Madison, University of Wisconsin Press, 1990.
16　J. Lewis, 'The Working-Class Wife and Mother and State Intervention, 1870–1918', in J. Lewis (ed.), *Labour and Love: Women's Experience of Home and Family, 1850-1940*, Oxford, Blackwell, 1986.
17　N. Sokoloff, *Between Money and Love. The Dialectics of Women's Home and Market Work*, New York, Praeger, 1980; C. Pateman, 'Feminist Critiques of the Public/Private Dichotomy', in C. Pateman (ed.), *The Disorder of Women*, Stanford, Stanford University Press, 1989.
18　C. Pateman, 'The Patriarchal Welfare State', in A. Gutman (ed.), *Democracy and the Welfare State*, Princeton, Princeton University Press, 1988.
19　S. M. Okin, *Women in Western Political Thought*, Princeton, Princeton University Press, 1979.
20　E. West, *Education and the State*, London, Institute of Economic Affairs, 1965; T. Parsons, and R. F. Bales, *Family Socialisation and Interaction Process*, Glencoe, Ill., Free Press, 1955.
21　M. Anderson, 'What is New about the Modern Family: A Historical Perspective', in British Society for Population Studies, *The Family*, London, OPCS, 1983.
22　R. Humphreys, 'The Poor Law and Charity. The COS in the

Provinces, 1870-1890', unpublished PhD thesis, University of London, 1991.

23 F. K. Prochaska, *Women and Philanthropy in Nineteenth-Century England*, Oxford, Clarendon Press, 1980.

24 P. Thane, 'Government and Society in England and Wales, 1750–1914', in F. M. L. Thompson (ed.), *The Cambridge Social History of Britain, 1750-1950*, vol. 3, *Social Agencies and Institutions*, Cambridge, Cambridge University Press, 1990.

25 J. Harris, 'Society and the State in Twentieth Century Britain', in F. M. L. Thompson (ed.), *The Cambridge Social History of Britain, 1750–1950*, vol. 3, *Social Agencies and Institutions*, Cambridge, Cambridge University Press, 1990.

26 E. Roberts, *A Woman's Place. An Oral History of Working Class Women*, Oxford, Blackwell, 1984.

27 F. Y. Edgeworth, 'Equal Pay to Men and Women for Equal Work', *Economic Journal*, 1922, vol. 32, p. 453.

28 COS, *Report of a Sub-Committee on House to House Visitation*, London, COS, 1870.

29 O. Hill, *Our Common Land*, London, Macmillan, 1877, p. 60.

30 O. Hill, *The Charity Organisation Society*, Occasional Paper, no. 15. London, COS, 1889.

31 E. Maurice (ed.), *Octavia Hill: Early Ideals*, London, Allen & Unwin, 1928, p. 211.

32 O. Hill, 'Organised Work among the Poor. Suggestions Founded on four Years' Management of a London Court', *Macmillans*, 1869, vol. 20, p. 222.

33 H. Mitchell, *The Hard Way Up*, London, Virago, 1977.

34 P. Thane, 'The Working Class and State "Welfare" in Britain, 1880–1914', *Historical Journal*, 1984, vol. 27.

35 J. Lee, 'The Integrity of the Family: A Vital Issue', COS Report, Bosanquet papers, Trunk II, Box H., n.d. Newcastle University Library.

36 V. Markham, 'The Problem of Poverty', *The Spectator*, 26 August 1911.

37 A. Martin, *Married Working Women*, London, National Union of Women's Suffrage Societies, 1911.

38 Fabian Women's Group, *How the National Insurance Bill affects Women*, London, FWG, 1911.

39 Women's Industrial Council, 'Memo on the National Insurance Bill as it affects Women', 1911, TS, BLPES, LSE.

40 *Report of the Departmental Committee on Sickness Benefit Claims under the National Insurance Act*, Cd. 7687, PP 1914–16, XXX, 1.

41 P. Thane, 'Women and the Poor Law in Victorian and Edwardian England', *History Workshop Journal*, 1978, no. 6.

42 *Report of the Royal Commission on the Poor Laws and the Relief of Distress*, Cd. 4499, PP 1909, XXXVII, 1.

43 *Report of the Proceedings of the National Conference on Infant Mortality, 1906*.

44 J. Lewis and C. Davies, 'Protective Legislation in Britain, 1870–1990:

Equality, Difference and their Implications for Women', *Policy and Politics*, 1991, vol. 19, no. 1.

45 *Final Report of the Treasury Committee on Civil Service Recruitment after War*, Cmd. 164, PP 1919, XI, 191.

46 *Report of the Committee on Social Insurance and Allied Services*, Cmd 6404, PP 1942, VI.

47 T. Skocpol and G. Ritter, 'Gender and the Origins of Modern Social Policies in Britain and the United States', *Studies in American Political Development*, 1991, vol. V (Spring); P. Baker, 'The Domestication of Politics: Women in American Political Society, 1780–1920', *American Historical Review*, 1984, vol. LXXXIX, no. 3; P Hollis, *Ladies Elect: Women in English Local Government, 1865–1914*, Oxford, Clarendon Press, 1987; S. Koven and S. Michel, 'Womanly Duties: Maternalist Politics and the Origins of Welfare States in France, Germany, Great Britain and the United States, 1880–1920', *American Historical Review*, 1990, vol. XCV, no. 4.

48 Wilensky and Lebaux, *Industrial Society*; P. Baldwin, *The Politics of Social Solidarity, Class Bases in the European Welfare State, 1875–1975*, Cambridge, Cambridge University Press, 1990; P. Evans, D. Rueschemeyer and T. Skocpol (eds), *Bringing the State Back In*, Cambridge, Cambridge University Press, 1985; R. Hay, 'Employers and Social Policy in Britain: The Evolution of Welfare Legislation, 1905–1914', *Social History*, 1977, vol. 4, no. 1.

49 K. Kish Sklar, 'The Historical foundations of Women's Power in the Creation of the American Welfare State, 1830-1930', in Seth Koven and Sonya Michel (eds), *Mothers of a New World. Maternalist Politics and the Origins of Welfare States*, London, Routledge, 1993.

50 Koven and Michel, 'Womanly Duties'.

51 Skocpol and Ritter, 'Gender and the Origins of Modern Social Policies'.

52 Thane, 'Government and Society'.

53 Hollis, *Ladies Elect*; Baker, 'Domestication of Politics'.

54 Hollis, *Ladies Elect*, p. 285.

55 P. Hall, H. Land, R. Parker and A. Webb, *Change, Choice and conflict in Social Policy*, London, Heinemann, 1975; J. Lewis, *The Politics of Motherhood. Child and Maternal Welfare in England, 1900–1939*, London, Croom Helm, 1980.

56 S. Pedersen, 'The Failure of Feminism in the Making of the British Welfare State'. *Radical History Review*, 1989, vol. XLIII.

57 J. Macnicol, *The English Movement for Family Allowances*, London, Heinemann, 1980.

58 Prochaska, *Women and Philanthropy*.

59 J. Lewis, *Women and Social Action in Victorian and Edwardian England*, Aldershot, Edward Elgar, 1991.

60 D. Riley, *'Am I that Name?' Feminism and the Category of 'Women' in History*, London, Macmillan, 1988.

Index

abortion 48, 60, 148, 165n47
Addison, Paul 188n42
age 25, 199, 205; *see also* child
  welfare; old age welfare
Alberti, J. 29n52
Aldrich Blake, Louisa 79
Allen, Marjory 151
Andersen, G. Esping 211
Anderson, Elizabeth Garrett 77,
  79, 88n63
Annan, Noel 93
annuities, old age 195
Anomalies Act (1931) 71, 220
anti-suffragists 10, 97–8, 108
Artisans' Dwelling Acts 118n12
Association of Head Mistresses
  17
Associations of Registered
  Medical Women 80
Atlantic Charter 5

Baker, Paula 222
Barnett, Henrietta 101, 102, 103,
  115, 116
Barnett, Samuel 102, 103, 115
Baylis, Lilian 113
Beale, Miss 17
Bell, E. Moberley 112
Bell, Mrs Harrison 158
Bentham, Ethel 157
Bentham, Jeremy 100
Benthamite ideology 2
Bevan, Aneurin 82
Beveridge, William 2, 3, 5, 71

Beveridge Report (1942) 5, 21,
  22, 23, 81, 183, 202–5, 220
birth control 16, 83, 143–66, 225;
  Meiji Japan 41, 48
Blake, Matilda 72
Boarding Out Society 132
Bodichon, Barbara Leigh Smith
  100, 101
Bond, Edward 99, 107, 111
Bondfield, Margaret 12–13
Booth, Charles 100, 197, 215
Bosanquet, Helen 29n51, 96, 215
Bowley, Sir Arthur Lyon 215
Brabazon occupational therapy
  scheme 131, 132
Braddock, Bessie 8
Briggs, A. 31n84
British Medical Association 77;
  1939 Nutrition Conference 173,
  179
Brittain, Vera 85
Brockway, Fenner 174
Browne, Stella 144, 152
Burdett Coutts, Angela 131
Burns, John 219
Buss, Miss 17

Canada 21–2
carers, women as 18–19, 71, 98–9,
  193, 201, 203, 204, 209, 211,
  215, 223
Carroll, Ethel 152
Chadwick, Edwin 100
charities 69

charity 9, 19, 213–14, 216, 217;
Louisa Twining and 125, 133–6,
137; and poor relief 193, 195,
213; *see also* voluntarism
Charity Organisation Society
(COS) 96, 97, 100, 103, 130–1,
133, 215, 217, 223
child allowances *see* family
allowances
child welfare 7, 13, 195, 213, 222;
health 4, 168, 176–80, 213;
Labour Party and 21, 167–88;
poverty 22, 172, 175, 176, 179;
see also maternity and child
welfare centres
childcare facilities 21, 213
Children First! (Labour Party)
167, 178
Children's Charter, (Labour Party)
167, 173, 181
Christian Socialism 100, 123
Churchill, Sir Winston 80
citizenship: of contribution 9–14,
84, 98–9, 224; gendered 9–14,
67–8, 83–4, 98, 209, 224; and
welfare state 23; *see also*
female agency; service
civil service 219–20, 222, 223;
pensions 196
Clark, Miss Murdoch 78
Coale, Ansley 60n3
Cobbe, Frances Power 29n50, 77,
138
Cockerell, Sidney 111
Cole, G.D.H. 167
collective biography 14–15, 94
collective self-help 9, 69–70
collectivism 3, 4; Labour Party
and child health and welfare
171–3, 180
community, local: care of elderly
poor in 190–4, 204; women's
suitability for work in 98
*Conference on the Giving of
Information on Birth Control
by Public Health Authorities,* 4
April 1930 161
Conrad, Christoph 199
Cons, Emma 101, 102, 113–14, 116

Conservative Party 4, 5, 169, 176,
179
contraception *see* birth control
Cooper, Selena 73
Co-operative Guild 145
Co-operativism 100, 171

Dalton, Hugh 177
Daniels, Nurse 143
Darley, Gillian 99
Davenport-Hill sisters 103
Davies, Emily 11, 17, 100
deaconess movement 134
decommodification, gendered
meaning of 211
democracy, Labour Party, child
welfare and future of 182, 183
demography and life expectancy
in developing countries 35,
37–59
Denmark 198
dependency, gendered meaning of
211
Dicey, A.V. 3
disability benefits/pensions 82,
195–6, 198
district nurses 124, 130, 140n15,
204
division of labour,
sexual/gendered 150, 151, 162,
198, 210, 211, 212, 223
divorce: Meiji Japan 46–7, 48, 52;
and provision of pensions 203,
204; Victorian 52
Donzelot, Jacques 63n29
Drake, Barbara 179
Ducie, Lady 103

Ecclesiastical Commissioners 96
economic development: and
excess female mortality 32–66;
and social welfare provision
6–8
economic recession/depression,
and welfare 22, 70–2, 78–9,
176–83
economics 3, 33, 35
Edgeworth, F.Y. 215
education 6, 10, 171, 213, 214,

222; Meiji Japan 42; Octavia
Hill and 97, 100, 101, 103; *see
also* schools
Eliot, George 99, 100, 101
Elshtain, J.B. 84
employment 22, 55; and old age
pension 196–8; pay for women
80, 134, 137, 223; philanthropy
as 122–42; of women 21, 84,
148, 201–2, 209–10, 212; *see
also* married women;
unemployment; work
equal compensation for personal
injuries 80
equal opportunities legislation 220
equal pay, campaign for 80, 223
equal-rights feminism 82, 83
eugenics, and birth control 145,
163n11
European Court of Justice ruling
on invalid care allowances for
married women 19
excess female mortality *see*
female mortality, excess

Fabian Women's Group 218
factory inspectors 222
Faderman, Lillian 109
family 1, 10, 11, 19, 24, 208, 223,
225; birth control and 152; and
care of elderly 191–2, 195;
Japanese 41, 46–53, 56–7,
59–60; Labour Party and 168–9,
182; male breadwinner model
13, 20–1, 208–10, 223, 225;
Octavia Hill and 98, 110; and
welfare state 23, 80–5, 203–5
family allowances 13, 15, 81, 83,
167, 170–3, 180, 181, 223
female agency 1, 14–21, 68, 72–4,
126–8, 202, 221; *see also*
citizenship; women, as
consumers/providers of welfare
female mortality, excess 32–66:
during development in Meiji
Japan 36–60; England and
Wales 32, 54–9; international
comparisons 38–41, 42, 43, 58
feminism *see* welfare feminism;

women's movement
feminist theory/thought 11, 20, 23,
67–8, 93, 208, 209
fertility, effects of state policies
36–60, 62n25
Finlayson, Geoffrey 9
France 8, 13, 221
Fraser, Andrew 62n28
friendly societies 75, 195, 196
friendly visiting 216–17, 223, 224;
see also social work
Furniss, Averil 170

Garrett Anderson, Elizabeth 77,
79, 88n63
gender: significance of 24–5,
167–8, 182, 208–10; and welfare
regimes 210–14; *see also* women
gender equality/inequality, of
welfare state 23–4, 203–4
gender politics 67–90
gender relations in Labour Party
154–6, 162, 181, 182, 223
gender roles 208, 215; and social
security system 203–4; *see also*
family, male breadwinner model
geriatrics 204
Germany 7, 12, 13, 198, 221
GFS 131, 132
Gibson, George 173
Girl's Friendly Society (GFS) 131,
132
Glasier, Katharine Bruce 175
Gooby, Peter Taylor 10
Gordon, Linda 151
Gould, Barbara Ayrton 170
Graves, Pamela 85, 163n8, 180,
185n14

Hall, Ruth 163n11
Harris, José 188n42
Harrison, B. 29n53
Hart, Ernest 103
Hastings, Somerville 171–2, 178,
179, 181
health 70, 75–80, 82, 147–8, 149;
Japan 49, 53; *see also* National
Health Insurance Scheme;
National Health Service

health care workers 84, 133, 204;
    see also nursing
*Health of the Nation: Why Are
    We C.3?* (Labour Party) 177–8
Henderson, Arthur 159, 184n12
Hill, Caroline 100, 106, 112
Hill, Emily 100, 112
Hill, Florence 112, 114
Hill, Gertrude 100, 112
Hill, James 99
Hill, Miranda 98, 112–13, 116
Hill, Octavia 2, 11, 16, 18,
    29nn50–1, 91–121, 132, 216
Hogg, Anna 103
Hollis, Patricia 11, 73, 131, 222,
    224
Holocaust 35
hospital boards 127
housing 6, 16, 18, 91–121, 148
Howell, David 188n42
Howitt, Mary 101
Hughes, Thomas 100
humanitarianism 168
Humphreys, R. 213
Humphries, Jane 65n78

Independent Labour Party (ILP)
    147, 171
Indian subcontinent 33–4, 39, 41,
    42, 43, 56
individualism, Japanese
    government and 53
inequality 209; *see also* gender
infant welfare *see* child welfare
infanticide 41–2, 46, 48, 54
intellectual climate, and formation
    of welfare state 3
international affairs, influence on
    welfare provision 175–6, 214;
    see also war
international comparisons: excess
    female mortality 38–41, 42, 43,
    58; old age pensions 198;
    welfare provision 6–8, 11–12,
    13, 21–2
International Council of Women
    202
international issue, welfare as:
    conferences on labour

    protection 7; women's
    campaigns 202
International Labour
    Organisation 8, 202, 219
Ishirara, Osamu 51
Italy 12, 67

Jameson, Anna 127
Jannetta, Ann B. 44, 45
Japan: excess female mortality
    during development 32–66;
    influence of Victorian England
    on management of women 6,
    52–3, 54
Jefferey, Miss 102
Jeffreys, Sheila 109–10
Jewson, Dorothy 149, 151, 155,
    158
Jex-Blake, Sophia 104–10
Johnston, Thomas 176
Jones, Helen 75

Kenney, Annie 116
Keynesianism 2, 3, 5, 21, 22, 183
Kingsley, Charles 99
Klasen, Stephen 60n3
Kolberg, J.E. 211
Koven, S. 11, 83, 221, 224
Kyrle Society 112, 131

labour legislation/protection 7, 12,
    16, 221
labour market: and child welfare
    168; in Japan 50–1, 58; gender
    and 19, 33–4, 80, 209–10; *see
    also* employment
Labour Party 2, 3, 4, 5, 6, 7, 84,
    200, 223; and birth control
    144–62; and child welfare 21,
    167–88; Conferences 147, 148,
    154–5, 157, 158, 159
Labour Woman, The 146, 147,
    152, 156, 157, 159, 170, 172,
    174, 177, 179, 182
Labour women 14, 74, 85: and
    birth control 145–62; and child
    welfare 167–82 *passim*
Ladies Guild 94
Langham Place Circle 17

Lansbury, George 70
Laski, Frida 151, 157
Last, Nella 81
Lawrence, Susan 174, 179
Lawther, Mrs 148
League of Nations 202
Lee, Jennie 171
Lee, Joseph 217
Leibfried, S. 211
lesbianism 109–10
Levine, Philippa 93–4, 109
Lewes, Charles 99, 100
Lewis, Jane 10, 21, 29n51, 68,
    90n96, 97
local government 132, 190, 223;
    campaign for birth control and
    143–4, 160–1; and mother/child
    welfare 75, 173–5, 177, 180,
    181; and old age 189 (*see also*
    poor law); and welfare
    provision 1, 6, 7, 10–11, 83, 214,
    221, 222
local welfare provision 2; women
    in 6, 10–11, 19, 67–80, 84, 132,
    223
London County Council 132,
    174–5, 179, 180
London School of Medicine for
    Women 77
lone parenthood 20, 81, 204, 209,
    210, 219
lunatic asylums 127
Lyman, Richard 188n42

MacDonald, Ramsay 147, 170
McHenry, Dean 186n19
McMillan, Margaret 169, 222
Malleson, Joan 151
Malone, L. L'Estrange 151
Malthusian League 144, 145, 147
Malthusianism 2, 144, 145, 146,
    147, 154
Manchester Public Assistance
    Committee 73
Markham, Violet 29n51, 222
married women: benefits 20, 71–2,
    75–6, 81, 82, 199, 203, 211–12,
    215, 218, 220; as carers 19, 215,
    223 (*see also* carers, women as);

employment 71–2, 201, 209,
    212, 215, 219–20, 225; exclusion
    from professions 13, 78, 219;
    property rights 41, 47–8, 52, 59,
    97, 101
Marshall, Alfred 3
Martin, Anna 218
Martindale, Louisa 77
Marwick, Arthur 181
Marxists 23
maternal welfare 150, 155–6, 171;
    see also birth control;
    maternalism; maternity;
    motherhood
maternalism 12, 13, 24, 67, 68, 75,
    83–5, 220–1, 224, 225; *see also*
    welfare feminism
maternity and child welfare
    centres 12, 75, 83, 143, 223
maternity grants 81
maternity leave 12, 219
Matrimonial Causes Act (1857)
    52
Maurice, Edmund 99, 100
Maurice, Frederick Denison 99,
    100, 123
Maxton, James 186n20
media: Louisa Twining's use of
    133; and widows' pensions in
    USA 67
medical practice 23; women in 16,
    76–80, 127
Medical Women's Federation 80
*Medical Women's Federation
    Newsletter* 80
Medical Women's Journal 79–80
medicine 178–9
Mencius 34–5
Metropolitan Association for
    Befriending Young Servants
    (MABYS) 131, 132
Michel, S. 11, 83, 221, 224
middle-class values/culture 217,
    224
middle-class women 12, 122, 201,
    212
midwives, role in Meiji Japan 41
militarism *see* war
Mitchell, Hannah 70, 217

Moorhouse, Mrs 73–4
moral dimension of welfare 9–10
Morris, William 100
motherhood 150, 209; Labour
    attitudes to 150–1, 153, 161–2;
    see also married women;
    maternal welfare; maternity
Mother's Meetings 75, 123, 135
mutual aid 9, 69–70

National Assistance 204
National Birthday Trust 70
National Conference on Infant
    Mortality (1906) 219
national efficiency/health, child
    welfare and 4, 168, 175–80, 182,
    183, 195, 214, 220
National Federation of Housing
    Societies 91
National Health Insurance
    Scheme (1911) 7, 12–13, 75–6,
    78, 80, 198, 218
National Health Service 76, 81,
    82–3
National Health Service (Family
    Planning) Act (1967) 89n88
national insurance 198, 220;
    women and administration of
    222; see also National Health
    Insurance Scheme
National Insurance Act (1911) see
    National Health Insurance
    Scheme
national politics: and birth control
    campaign 143, 155, 156–60, 162;
    women's activity 74, 76, 81,
    84–5, 222–3
National Spinsters' Pensions
    Association 82, 201
National Trust 91, 96, 112
National Union of Societies for
    Equal Citizenship 166n7
networks, female 1, 7, 14–18; in
    housing 16, 91–121; Louisa
    Twining and philanthropic 128,
    129–33, 136; mutual aid 70;
    professional 72, 79–80
New Hospital for Women 79
New Liberalism 3, 5, 214, 221

New Right 22, 23
New Zealand 198
NHS (Family Planning) Act
    (1967) 89n88
Nightingale, Florence 29n50, 97,
    100, 101, 135
Noel-Buxton, Lucy 175
Norway 7
nursing 122, 123, 124, 125, 128,
    129, 130, 131, 133, 134–6, 137,
    140n15
Nursing Notes 133
nutrition: children and 176–80;
    women 57, 70

Oakley, Ann 208
Octavia Hill Club 102
Okin, S.M. 213
old age: construction of 194, 199,
    204; in Japan 49–50; mortality
    ratios of Victorian England and
    Japan 57–8
old age welfare 123, 189–207, 213;
    aged poor in pre-industrial
    England 190–4; demand for old
    age pensions 194–9; insurance
    pensions and lowering of
    pension age for women
    199–202; international women's
    campaigns 202; system of
    Beveridge Report and after
    202–5
Open Spaces movement 96, 98,
    100
Organisation of Labour Women
    16, 150, 155, 156, 157, 159,
    162n2
Ottley, Alice 11
Owen, David 142n63

Parker, J. 29n50
Pateman, C. 212
paternalism 67, 221, 224
patriarchy: in Meiji Japan 44–5,
    47; public, of welfare policy
    205, 208–9; in South Asia 33–4
Pedersen, Susan 173, 182, 223
pensions see old age welfare;
    women

Pensions Act (1908) 199
philanthropy 9; case studies of
    Octavia Hill and Louisa
    Twining 91–142; *see also*
    charity; voluntarism
Phillips, Marion 147, 156, 157,
    159, 170–1
Phillpott, H.R.S. 174
philosophy 3, 212
physical fitness campaign 175
police force, used to enforce state
    policy in Meiji Japan 36, 41
Political and Economic Planning 3
political parties, and welfare
    policy 1, 5; *see also*
    Conservative Party; Labour
    Party
political system, changes in, and
    development of welfare state
    5–6
politics, national *see* national
    politics
poor law 20, 58, 83, 122, 124, 136,
    139, 190, 192–5, 197, 198, 219;
    gender politics 68–74; *see also*
    workhouse nursing; workhouses
Poor Law Acts 2, 204–5
poor law guardians 10–11, 18, 70,
    71, 72–4, 84, 112, 124, 129–30,
    132–3, 138, 139, 222
poor law inspectors 111
Potter, Beatrice *see* Webb,
    Beatrice
Potter, Catherine 102–3
poverty: female 68–74, 75, 192; of
    old people 58, 204; *see also*
    child welfare; poor law
poverty lobby 23
*Preserve the Real Wealth of the
    Nation* (Labour Party) 174
pressure groups, and welfare
    policy 1, 130, 190; *see also*
    voluntarism
Preston, S. 37, 38, 39, 40, 42, 44,
    45, 49, 51, 55, 62n23
prisons 127
Prochaska, F. 9
professionalisation of women's
    work 136–9

professions 13, 23, 171, 219; *see
    also* medical practice
property rights of women 57, 58,
    59, 60, 97, 101; in Meiji Japan
    41, 47–8; Victorian England 52,
    59
prosopography 14–15, 94
prostitution, Japanese 51, 65n67
Provision of Meals Act 177
public assistance committees 71
public health: policy 35, 43;
    women in 78, 222
public/private 14, 17, 190, 212;
    Louisa Twining and 122, 123–4,
    127, 131, 136; maternalism and
    24, 83–4; Octavia Hill and 97,
    115, 118

Quakers 93

race, and welfare 20, 205
racial degeneration/health *see*
    national efficiency/health
Rathbone, Eleanor 13, 15, 29n52,
    68, 171, 187n34
relief agencies 69, 96, 117; *see
    also* poor law; voluntarism
religion: Louisa Twining and 123,
    125, 137; and welfare 9
Rendall, Jane 93
Ritter, G. 221
romantic friendship 109–10
romantic love 59; Japan 53
Rose, H. 31n86
Rose, June 163n11
Rowbotham, Sheila 150
Rowe, Sir Reginald 91
Royal College of Physicians 77,
    78, 79
Royal Commission on National
    Health Insurance (1926) 75, 147
Royal Commission on the
    Housing of the Working
    Classes (1884) 96, 102
Royal Commission on the Poor
    Law 96, 219
Royal Institution 122
Ruskin, John 94, 99, 100, 107, 111
Russell, Dora 144, 148, 151, 152,

157, 158, 159, 162n2
Russell-Gurney, Mrs 103

St Luke's Home for Epileptic and
    Incurable Women 123
Salter, Alfred 171, 172, 178
Say, Jean-Baptiste 62n19
Scandinavia 12, 202; Denmark
    198; feminist thought 208;
    Norway 7; Sweden 8, 39–40, 42,
    43
Scharlieb, Mary 79, 152
schools 213; meals service 168,
    174, 175, 177, 178, 179, 180, 217,
    223; medical officers/services
    77–8, 167, 174, 175, 177, 178,
    217–18; see also education
scientism, Labour Party and child
    welfare 178–80, 182
Select Committee of the House
    of Lords on Metropolitan
    Hospitals (1891) 141n38
Select Committee on the
    Administration and Relief of
    the Poor (1861) 124
self-help 9, 69, 193
Sen, Amartya 60n3
Senior, Jane Nassau 100, 111
separated women 194; allowances
    203
service 136; see also citizenship, of
    contribution
settlement work 96, 97, 100
sexuality, attitudes to, as element
    in birth control campaign 144,
    145, 150, 151, 152–3, 154, 156,
    162
Shaen, William 103
Shaftesbury, Lord 99, 100
Shorter, Edward 61n7
single parenthood 20, 81, 204,
    209, 210, 219
single women 210; benefits 82,
    200–2, 203
SJCIWO 165n60, 170, 178, 180,
    181
Sklar, Kathryn Kish 220
Skocpol, T. 12, 221, 224
SMA 174, 178, 180, 181, 182

Smiles, Samuel 69
Smith, Gladys Miall 78
Smith, H.L. 80
Smith, Robert 63n34
Smith, Southward 100
smoke-abatement 100
Snell, Lord 179
Snowden, Philip 168
social change 10, 224
social class 16, 20, 24, 25, 205,
    208, 220; and birth control 144,
    145, 149, 163n6; and child
    health 176–7; and excess female
    mortality 58–9; and family
    allowances 171; Labour Party
    and welfare 74, 83, 84, 117, 147;
    and patriarchy in Japan 44–5,
    47; see also middle class;
    working class
social feminists 7
social insurance 7, 8, 198; see also
    national insurance; National
    Health Insurance Scheme
social justice 2
social order 193
Social Science Association 140n13
social security system 23, 202–4,
    212, 220; see also old age
    welfare; unemployment
social services 6, 204
social surveys 176
social theory 212
social work 10, 190, 216, 221, 224;
    training for 96; see also friendly
    visiting
socialism 5, 7; and child health
    168, 169, 175; Worker's Birth
    Control Group and 147–9, 153,
    158, 160
Socialist Doctor, The 178
Socialist Medical Association
    (SMA) 174, 178, 180, 181, 182
Society for Constructive Birth
    Control and Racial Progress
    145
Society for the Provision of Birth
    Control Clinics 166n72
Society of Women Housing
    Managers 96, 102

sociology, and excess female
    mortality 33–4, 35
Sokoloff, N. 212
South Asia 33–4, 39, 41, 42, 43,
    56
Soviet Union 8
Spencer, Herbert 212
spinsters see single women
Standing Joint Committee of
    Industrial Women's
    Organisations (SJCIWO)
    165n60, 170, 178, 180, 181
Stanley, Liz 93, 101
Stansfield, Lord 111
state: and birth control provision
    143–4, 161–2; and excess female
    mortality during development
    33, 34–60; provision of old age
    pensions 197–205; role of 1–2,
    8, 15, 21, 22, 208, 213–14, 216,
    217, 221, 223–4 (in provision of
    workhouse nurses 135–6, 137);
    policy 67, 202, 214, 225
Staves, Susan 59
Stedman-Jones, Gareth 118n12
Stephen, Sir Lesley 100
Sterling sisters 103
Stopes, Marie 144, 145, 147
Strachey, Ray 29n52, 93
Strand Union 124–5
Sturge, Elizabeth 103
suffragette movement 116
Summerfield, P. 14
Sutherland, Mary 168, 175
Sweden 8; excess female mortality
    39–40, 42, 43

Tabutin, Dominique 64n42
Taunton Commission on
    secondary schooling (1865) 17
Temperance Societies 135
textile industry, women's
    employment in 50–1, 58, 72
Thane, P. 14, 74, 173, 180, 191,
    214, 217
Thatcherism 22
Thurtle, Ernest 143, 148, 155
Titmuss, R. 23, 208, 211
Todd, Margaret 109, 110

Townsend, Miss 115
trade unions 171, 182, 195, 196,
    197, 223; see also TUC
tuberculosis 57
TUC 170, 171, 172–3, 177
Turner, Lillie 146
Tweedie, Jill 115
Twining, Elizabeth 123
Twining, Louisa 10–11, 18, 29n50,
    122–42

unemployment 8, 26n14, 179, 199;
    see also employment
unemployment insurance 8,
    12–13, 71, 76, 198, 212, 218, 220
UNICEF 61n10
Unitarians 93
United States 7, 12, 13, 20, 67,
    212, 220–1, 222; excess female
    mortality 58, 59
unmarried mothers 81, 219; see
    also single parenthood
unmarried women 210; benefits
    82, 200–2, 203

Vicinus, Martha 17, 93
voluntarism 1, 2, 7, 8–13, 22, 67,
    208, 213–14, 220, 221, 223–4,
    225; birth control clinics 144,
    145, 146; Louisa Twining and
    130–6, 138; and old age 190; see
    also philanthropy

war: and formation of welfare
    state 3–5, 7, 14, 21, 175–6; and
    welfare policy in Meiji Japan
    46, 51–3, 59; women in wartime
    14, 21, 80, 81
Ward, Mrs Humphry 222
Ward, L. 163n6
Warren, Marjorie 204
Webb, Beatrice 8, 29nn50–1, 96,
    100, 103, 116, 174, 222
Webb, Sidney 8
Webster, Charles 188n42
welfare: gender and see gender;
    as mixed economy in Britain 2,
    8, 22, 208, 210–14, 221–2
welfare dependency 71, 211

welfare development, history of: before classic welfare state 1–8, 212; forms of female agency 14–21; gendered contribution to welfare 8–14, 220–5; welfare state onwards 21–5
welfare feminism 7, 13, 15, 68, 75, 80, 81–2, 83, 170–1, 202, 223; and birth control campaign 144, 147, 149–54, 162, 163n6
welfare policy 1, 208, 214; women's influence on *see* female agency; networks; *see also* Labour Party; state
welfare state, classic 8, 21–5, 68, 80–5, 202–5, 220, 224
Welshman, John 176
WGS 72, 124, 131, 132
White, Florence 82
widows: pensions/benefits 67, 81, 82, 200; and poor law 194, 195, 219; position in Meiji Japan 41
Wilkinson, Ellen 159, 176–7
Williams, Mrs Theodore 132
Wilson, Jane 131
Wiswell, Ella Lury 63n34
Witcop-Aldred, Rose 151, 156
women: and child welfare 167–8, 169–75; as consumers/providers of welfare 1, 5–6, 23, 168, 169 (as clients 19–21, 68–72, 75–6, as providers 8–14, 72–4, 76–80, 213, 220–5); enfranchisement and political involvement 5–6, 7, 15, 83–5, 97–8, 169; mid-Victorian 54–9; pensions 67, 81, 82, 83, 134, 194, 198–204, 221; and state policy in Meiji Japan 41–59, 76; in wartime 14, 21, 80, 81; *see also* female agency; Labour women; married women
Women and the General Election (Labour Party) 170
Women in Local Government Society (WLGS) 124, 131, 132, 138
women MPs 76, 81
Women's Co-operative Guild 163n6, 181
Women's Freedom League 82
women's groups *see* welfare feminism; women's movement
Women's Guardians Society (WGS) 72, 124, 131, 132
women's history 122
Women's Industrial Council 13, 218
Women's Local Government Association 222
women's movement 9–10, 15–16, 67, 76–7, 82, 93–4, 109, 200, 203; in Japan 41, 47, 53, 56; Octavia Hill and 97, 104; *see also* networks; welfare feminism
Women's National Liberal Federation 166n72
Women's University Settlement 96, 100
work 115, 193; paid and unpaid, and welfare 13, 210–11; professionalisation of women's 136–9; *see also* employment
Worker's Birth Control Group (WBCG) 16, 144–62, 162n2, 163n6, 166n72; campaign in the Labour Party 154–60; and feminism 149–54, 158, 160; and socialism 147–9, 153, 158, 160
Workhouse Girls Aid Committee 131
workhouse nursing 122, 123, 124, 128, 129, 130, 134–6, 137
Workhouse Nursing Association (WNA) 124, 130, 132, 133, 134, 135, 138, 139
Workhouse Visiting Society (WVS) 124, 130, 139
Workhouse Visiting Society's Industrial Home 123
workhouses 10–11, 20, 111, 123, 124–5, 126–7, 195, 222; *see also* poor law; workhouse nursing
working class 5, 6, 7; and old age pensions 194; *see also* housing
working-class movements 24
working-class women 54, 215–16; and birth control campaign 16,144–62; employment 201,

212, 215; as poor law guardians 72, 73
Working Men's College 100, 103
World League for Sexual Reform 152
World War I 4, 75, 79, 81, 177, 201, 223
World War II 4–5, 8, 79, 80, 81, 183, 212
Worthing District Nursing Committee 125, 130, 135

Yamada, Waka 47
Yorke, Harriot 111–12
Young, Andrew 169
youth work 100

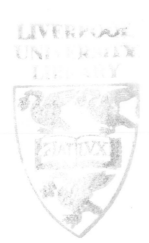